A PATIENT'S GUIDE TO LIPOSUCTION

How to Make an Informed Decision

JEFFRY B. SCHAFER, MD, FRSM

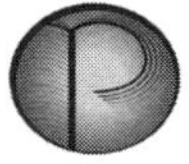

Outskirts Press, Inc.
Denver, Colorado

A Patient's Guide to Liposuction
How to Make an Informed Decision
All Rights Reserved.
Copyright © 2011 Jeffry B. Schafer, M.D., FRSM
v2.0

Cover Photo © 2011 JupiterImages Corporation. All rights reserved - used with permission.

DISCLAIMER

Outskirts Press, Inc.
http://www.outskirtspress.com

ISBN: 978-1-4327-8147-7

Outskirts Press and the "OP" logo are trademarks belonging to Outskirts Press, Inc.

PRINTED IN THE UNITED STATES OF AMERICA

Dedication

This book is dedicated to my loving wife, Sandy,
our standard poodle daughter, Joelle,
and to all my mentors who have given their time to train me.

Acknowledgements

I would like to thank my extremely capable administrative and surgical staff at New Image Cosmetic Surgery: Kitty Buckley - Administrative Assistant, Alice Schultz – Medical Assistant, and Eliza Pangan – Office Receptionist.

Very special thanks to Tammy Ladderbush, my Surgical Consultant, for researching and preparing photos, and to Constance Hageman, who devoted countless hours editing data, graphics, and photos in preparation for publishing.

Contents

Introduction

COSMETIC SURGERY HAS changed dramatically since the 1980s. Technology has advanced, techniques have improved, and cosmetic procedures are safer than ever before.

Liposuction is one procedure that has advanced exponentially, because it quickly (and permanently) alters a patient's appearance. One day can literally change the rest of a person's life.

Men and women dissatisfied with body appearance — whether genetic or altered — often find that diet and exercise alone don't give them the shape and definition they desire.

Liposuction is my personal passion; you could say that I express my creativity by sculpting bodies.

There are many scientific publications and textbooks on liposuction. Most are presented in technical language meant for medical professionals, not for prospective patients.

I decided it was time to write a book that simplifies the subject and allows me to share my knowledge, expertise, and successes with those considering liposuction. This book will help patients understand the basics of liposuction and the results that can be achieved.

Over twenty-five years ago, I shifted the focus of my cosmetic surgery practice to liposuction. I've invested years studying textbooks and articles, learning from the great "masters" of liposuction. More importantly, I spent hours in operating rooms with these eminent doctors in order to study their techniques closely.

I had the honor of studying with Dr. Giorgio Fischer (known as the father of liposuction) and Dr. Pierre Fournier (inventor of the syringe technique of liposuction) when they lectured in Washington, D.C.

I was invited to operate alongside Dr. Marco Gasparotti, the inventor of superficial liposuction, in La Jolla, California.

I attended intensive operating room classes led by Dr. Jeffrey Klein of San Juan Capistrano, California, inventor of the "wet" technique of tumescent liposuction.

Liposuction is my chosen specialty, and I continually strive to perfect my techniques. I've gained a tremendous amount of experience, performing an average of 700 liposuction surgeries a year.

On the surface, this may not sound like many procedures but, on average, each patient wants to improve at least six areas of the body. So, in reality, I perform approximately 10,000 liposuction procedures on those 700 patients.

The Early Days of Liposuction

Liposuction was pioneered in France in the mid-1970s. Originally, it could only be afforded by the rich and famous, out of reach for the average person. Today, liposuction is one of the most commonly performed cosmetic procedures in the world.

Early on, liposuction was performed in a hospital setting under general anesthesia. The original cannulas used for suctioning were awkward blunt-tipped hollow tubes connected to a vacuum suction pump.

This surgery resulted in extensive bruising, substantial blood loss, and removed only small amounts of fat at a time. Understandably, this procedure wasn't immediately popular (or appealing).

The invention of the wet technique of liposuction by Dr. Jeffrey Klein in 1985 dramatically changed how liposuction was performed, and improved its image in the eyes of both medical professionals and the public.

Dr. Klein's technique used a mixture of the drugs lidocaine and epinephrine which, when combined, could anesthetize (numb) the area, constrict the blood vessels, and inhibit bleeding.

This innovative procedure allowed the fat to be floated out in infused fluid, rather than via the patient's blood. Today, the tumescent technique is used in most liposuction procedures.

Dr. Klein's microcannulas were smaller in size and more efficient than the original cannulas. In November, 2006, even smaller cannulas were introduced with the advent of SmartLipo®.

According to Dr. Alberto Goldman, distinguished surgeon from Porto Alegre, Brazil, SmartLipo "employs laser energy in direct contact with fat and other tissues promoting the disruption of fat cells and, at the same time…stimulates the dermis with a consequent neo-collagen production resulting in skin tightening."

He further states that there is "potential improvement of areas of flaccidity in the body and face"…representing…"one of the most important effects related to this very new surgical option. Other important indications include the treatment of hyperhidrosis (excessive sweating in the arm pit area) and bromidrosis (body odor)."

Liposuction Today

Instruments and equipment for liposuction are constantly being improved. Many manufacturers rely on cosmetic surgery practices like mine for testing new technologies.

Being on the cutting edge in this rapidly expanding industry allows liposuction specialists to offer patients the most advanced, improved techniques available.

Why Write This Book?

My goal is to provide all the information currently available about liposuction. I'll answer common questions, address pertinent issues, and provide a basis to help patients make intelligent, informed liposuction choices.

Discussing cosmetic techniques and procedures with a surgeon can be intimidating, and a prospective patient may worry about asking the right questions.

I answer many of those questions in this book, giving all the information I have at my disposal in a format that's straightforward and easy to understand. I explain current surgical techniques and give you my objective opinions about their benefits and weaknesses.

I discuss how to select a surgeon and give you a list of questions to ask during the initial interview. You'll learn how different areas of the body respond to liposuction. Actual before-and-after photos will help you form realistic expectations of what liposuction can and can't do.

Understanding Liposuction

Anticipating any surgery can cause anxiety. Understanding liposuction procedures can be invaluable, and alleviate that concern. I'll explain everything from preparing for surgery to recovering as rapidly as possible.

You'll see photographs of patients, from the day of surgery through the ensuing weeks. These show you what to expect before and after the procedure. There's also a guideline to help you determine when you may safely return to pre-surgical activities.

What about Complications?

Many patients worry about complications, or what could go wrong. I devote an entire chapter to putting those concerns into perspective.

Realistically speaking, there *have* been unsatisfactory outcomes in liposuction, as with any surgical procedures. In this book I'll give you the tools to select the most qualified and experienced surgeon, so the risk of complications will be minimal.

1

Liposuction and How It Works

LIPOSUCTION GENTLY REMOVES a portion of fat cells from localized areas of the body, while preserving nerves, blood vessels, and connective tissue. A blunt-tipped cannula attached to a suction device removes the cells, which are then vacuumed out of the tissue, suspended in a sterile solution.

Fat Cells

Fat provides fuel for the body. Ironically, the most common sites of unwanted fat are precisely the areas that have an affinity for fat accumulation; any fat available in the blood stream is quickly appropriated by these cells.

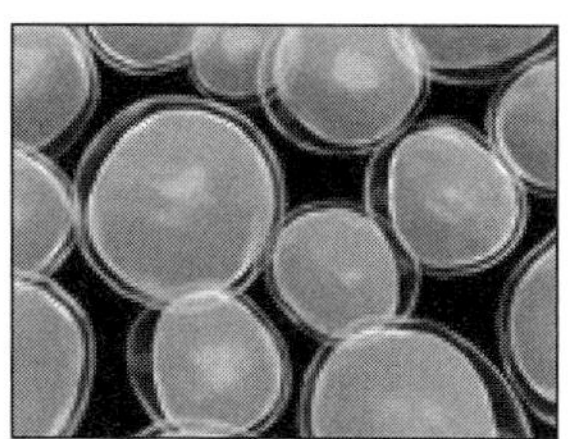

FIGURE 1-1
HUMAN FAT CELLS

The location and abundance of fat cells within the body determine a person's overall shape and appearance, although body structure is also influenced by heredity.

Individuals are born with a certain number of fat cells and, as weight is gained or lost, these cells can expand or shrink. Figure 1-1 is a picture of human adipocytes (fat cells).

There's no way to control fat deposits since they're resistant to diet and exercise. The only way to permanently eliminate fat is through liposuction. Consequently, liposuction has become one of the most commonly-performed cosmetic surgery procedures in the world.

Weight Gain

With age, metabolism decreases, so it's necessary to either increase exercise and/or decrease dietary intake to maintain a healthy weight.

It's a myth that fat cells increase when a significant amount of weight is gained. The amount of cells remains constant. Weight gain simply enlarges those cells. After liposuction, fat cells in other areas can expand, but the patient won't grow new cells where liposuction was performed.

Skin Irregularities

Patients frequently ask if liposuction can correct irregularities of the skin. Liposuction may *improve* dimpled or wrinkled skin, but not correct it. Smartlipo® is a great improvement over previous methods of liposuction, and can tighten the skin and smooth wrinkles. Areas of cellulite may also be improved with liposuction, sometimes significantly.

My Introduction to SmartLipo®

Ironically, I first read about the newly-introduced *SmartLipo* in People® magazine. I contacted the manufacturing company, Cynosure, and was invited to fly to Boca Raton, Florida, to study with Dr. Alberto

Goldman, foremost researcher and author of numerous SmartLipo publications.

Liposculpture vs Liposuction

The difference between liposculpture and liposuction is the degree of body-contouring and shaping achieved. Liposuction simply removes fat.

Liposculpture is a refined liposuction technique that produces more precise results, actually improving the shape of the treated area. I have performed thousands of liposculpture procedures.

Body Contouring vs Weight Loss

Ironically, even tri-athletes and U.S. Navy Seals (who are optimally fit), can have areas of unwanted fat. When diet and exercise are ineffective, liposuction can be beneficial. But liposuction was developed for body contouring, not weight loss.

After undergoing liposuction, a patient may have a greater incentive to exercise, in order to see further improvement. Some patients even say that liposuction gave them a jump-start to take better care of themselves, by starting and sticking to workout regimes.

Liposuction

The tumescent technique of liposuction introduces fluid into the target area. This fluid has several components, including:

- Saline solution which aids in fat removal
- Lidocaine, an anesthetic medication that reduces pain during and after a procedure. A patient's weight determines how much lidocaine is used
- Epinephrine, a medication which constricts blood vessels to inhibit bleeding

The use of these medications limits blood and body-fluid loss, making liposuction safer and less painful than ever before. Bruising is minimized in the liposuction target area, resulting in a quicker return to normal for the patient.

A surgeon must limit the area and amount of fat suctioned in one session. As safe as the tumescent technique is, it still causes some blood loss, and carries the possibility of lidocaine toxicity.

Some surgeons won't remove more than 3 or 4 liters of material in one session, including fat, blood, and infiltrated fluids. Other doctors measure only the fat, and may remove up to 5 liters of material*.

*Removing over 6 liters of fat is considered *mega-lipo,* and must be done in a hospital setting.

Drastic fat and fluid removal can trigger blood chemistry to change, causing it to fall to unsafe levels, threatening the patient's safety.

When liposuction is performed correctly, there should be no significant blood loss or anesthetic toxicity. In fact, the blood lost when the lab specimen is drawn is usually greater than what's lost during the entire surgical procedure.

Pre-Operative Lab Work

Prior to surgery, you'll have lab tests, including one that shows levels of hemoglobin (the protein in red blood cells) and hematocrit (the proportion of red blood cells present). These tests help determine if you have anemia or an active infection.

Some surgeons also request a coagulation panel. This test shows the ability of your blood to clot normally. That's an important factor in reducing intra- and post-operative bleeding and bruising. Finally, many surgeons require an HIV test prior to surgery.

These pre-operative blood tests and panels give the surgeon a current benchmark of the patient's overall health, to ensure the procedure can be performed safely, with the least chance of complications.

Questionable lab results should be addressed by the ordering physician prior to surgery.

Anesthesia

As I mentioned earlier, an anesthetic makes the patient comfortable during the liposuction procedure. The type of anesthesia to be used is chosen by the surgeon.

Some physicians prefer "twilight" (conscious) sedation while others require general anesthesia. General anesthesia paralyzes the patient's breathing, with a tube placed in the throat connected to a machine that takes over respiration. General anesthesia can result in nausea and vomiting, cardiac irregularities, and other significant side effects.

My personal feeling is that the use of general anesthesia is unnecessary, and that safer alternatives (such as the aforementioned twilight anesthesia) or oral sedation, when administered by a skilled practitioner, provide the most comfortable experience for a patient.

Post-Operative Garments

Post-operative garments are essential during the healing process. Liposuction patients are placed in compression garments post-procedure, which vary depending on the areas of the body treated.

These garments provide constant and steady compression in order to reduce swelling and bruising. They can also smooth out the tissue, providing optimal results.

The garment must extend above and below areas treated (e.g. for inner thighs, garment needs to extend down the leg to below the knees). Figure 1-2 shows some common post-op garments.

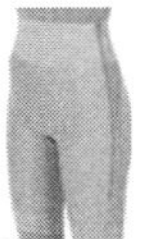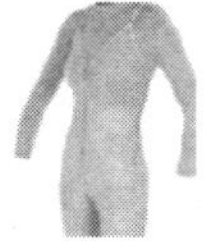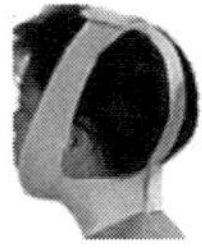

FIGURE 1-2
COMPRESSION GARMENTS

Better techniques and improved understanding of post-op recovery now allow patients to change into a second-stage garment after several days. For example, in post-op abdominal procedures, the patient will be dressed in an abdominal binder. Secondary garments are less restrictive, more like panty hose.

You may purchase secondary garments known as "body-shapers" (e.g. Spanx®) at major department stores or online. Stores often carry their own brands of shapewear which provide adequate support during post-op healing.

Some department stores that carry recommended shapewear are:

- Kohl's   (Flexees®, Jockey®)
- Macy's   (Flexees)
- Nordstrom   (Spanx)
- Target   (Assets®)

These specialty websites offer the finest in body-shaping garments:

- annette.com
- lipoinabox.com
- makemeheal.com

Liposuction Revisions

Patients are often concerned about the possibility of revisions or corrections after liposuction. It's not uncommon for a patient who underwent traditional liposuction to require a secondary procedure. The rate may be as high as 20 percent of procedures performed. But new technology has significantly decreased the need for revisions.

Even a procedure performed by an experienced practitioner can result in residual fat or a depression in the target area.

Before undergoing liposuction, a patient should recognize the possibility of a secondary procedure.

Imperfections, not seen initially due to swelling after the procedure, can be corrected after four to six months, the recommended length of time for treated areas to resolve, following liposuction.

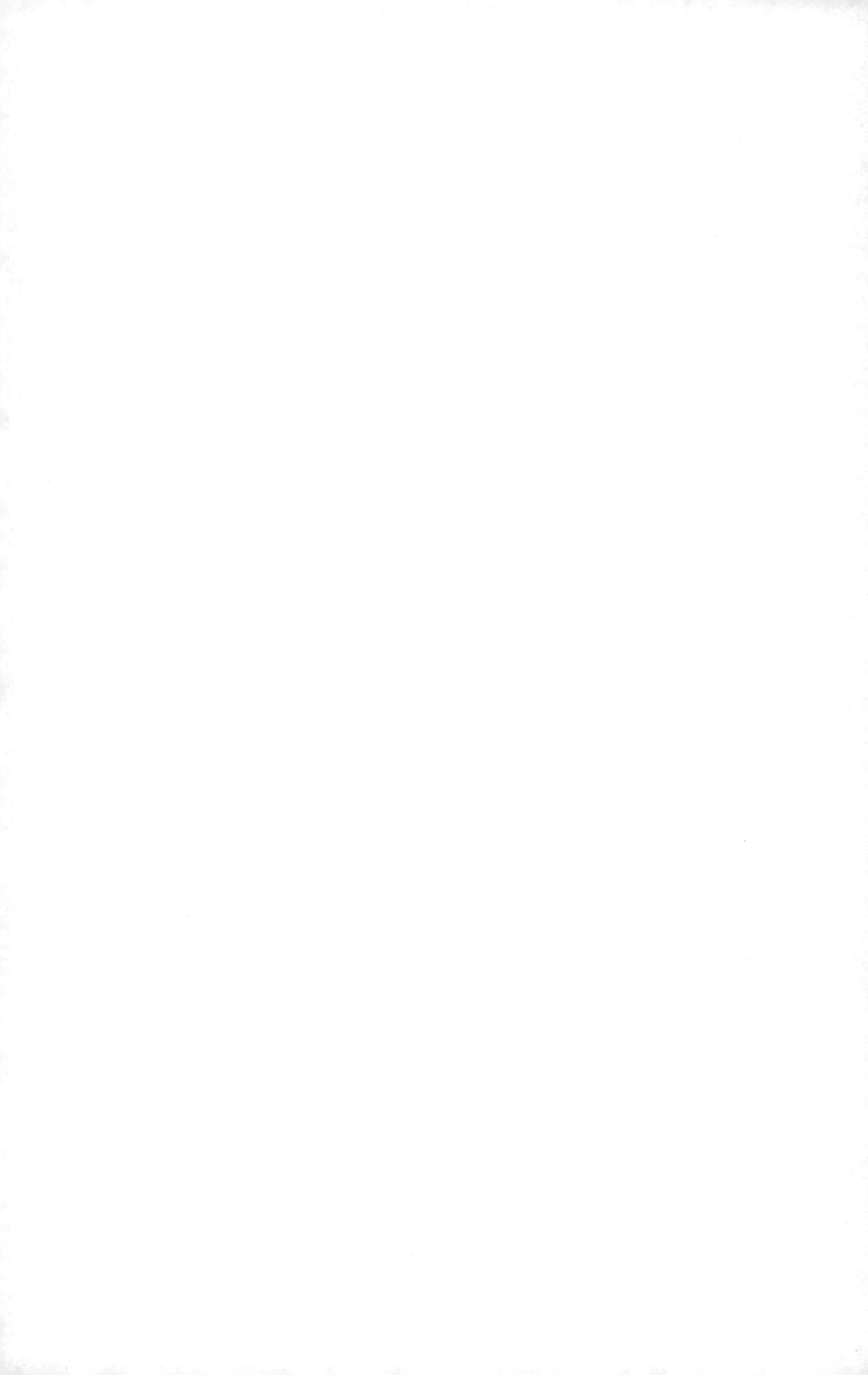

2

Am I a Good Candidate for Liposuction?

How to Make an Informed Decision

PATIENTS COMING TO me for liposuction usually range in age from twenty to sixty. Ideally, they're less than twenty pounds overweight, exercise regularly, and follow a healthy diet.

Younger patients have the best results because of their skin's elasticity. However, liposuction procedures benefit almost everyone, even those over the age of sixty. I've treated many patients in their seventies, with outstanding results.

Look at Figures 2-1 and 2-2.

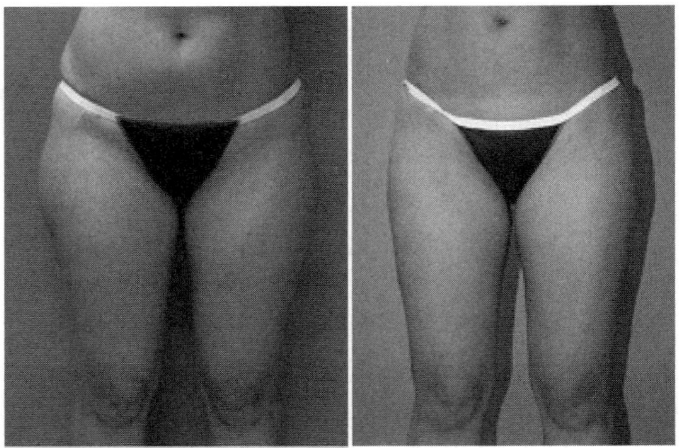

BEFORE   FIGURE 2-1   AFTER
ACTUAL 25-YEAR-OLD PATIENT

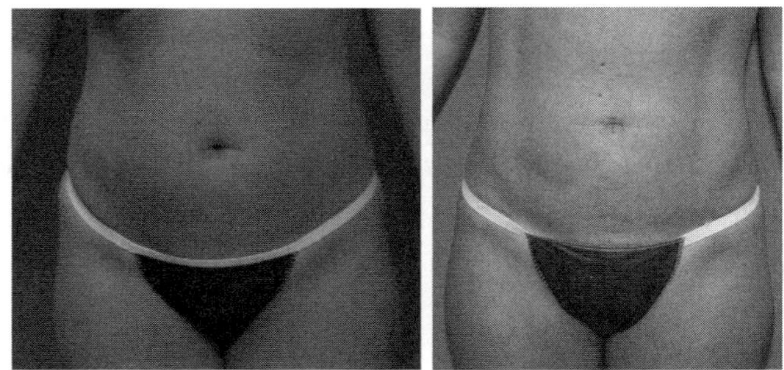

BEFORE   FIGURE 2-2   AFTER
ACTUAL 55-YEAR-OLD PATIENT

The age difference between these two patients is 30 years, but each was able to achieve substantial improvement following their liposuction procedures.

Liposuction Demographics

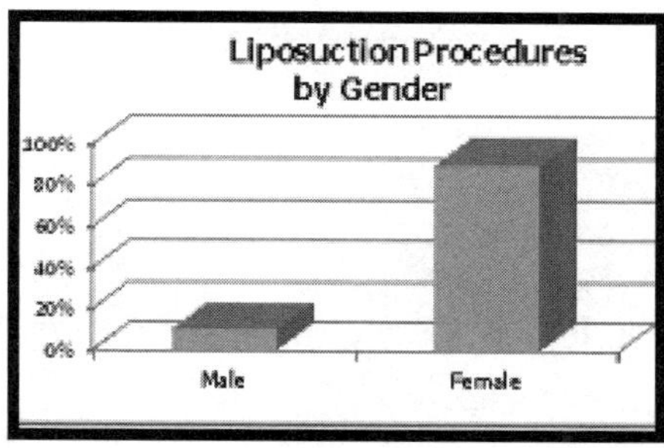

FIGURE 2-3
PROCEDURES BY GENDER

Today, staying youthful is critical in order to successfully compete in the business world.

As can be seen in Figure 2-3, the majority of liposuction procedures (90 percent) are performed on women.

This dynamic, however, is changing; more men are making the decision to "tweak" their faces and physiques, but don't want it to be obvious. My *Weekend Recovery®* makes it possible to have a cosmetic procedure on Friday and return to work on Monday, looking refreshed and rested.

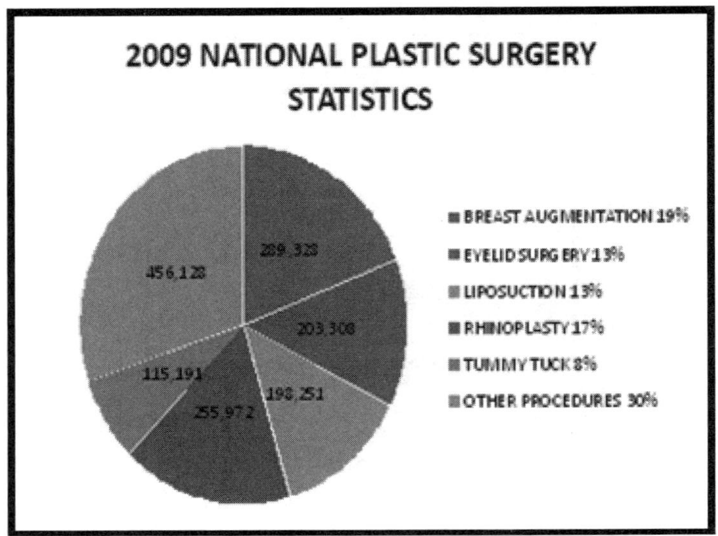

FIGURE 2-4
UNITED STATES PLASTIC SURGERY STATISTICS, 2009

It may be interesting to see what procedures are most popular in the United States. Figure 2-4 is a chart showing the cosmetic surgery statistics from 2009.

Body Mass Index (BMI)

BMI is a number calculated using a person's weight and height, and provides a reliable indicator of body fat for most adults 20 years old and up. BMI is interpreted using standard weight categories for both men and women. The lower these numbers are, the healthier the person, especially in terms of cardiovascular disease and diabetes.

BMI uses this formula:

BMI = weight (in lbs) divided by height (in inches^2) times 703*
* = CONVERSION FACTOR

Example: A person weighs 140 lbs and is 5'5" (65") tall.
           Calculation: [140 ÷ (65^2)] x 703 = 23.29

If your BMI is:

- less than 18.5, it falls within the "underweight" range
- 18.5 to 24.9, it falls within the "normal", or healthy, weight range
- 25.0 to 29.9, it falls within the "overweight" range
- 30.0 or higher, it falls within the "obese" range

The person in our example is within the normal range, at 23.29.

The terms obese and overweight describe ranges of weight that are greater than what's considered healthy for a given height, while underweight describes a weight that's lower than what's considered healthy.

BMI helps assess the health risk that an over- or under-weight patient faces, as seen in Figure 2-5 below. However, weight only tells you how hefty you are, not how healthy you are.

Belly fat can be an indicator of multiple medical problems. So included in the chart is a *Waist Size* calculator, another means of determining overweight and obesity.

Risk of Associated Disease According to BMI and Waist Size			
BMI		Waist = 40"(M) 35"(F)	Waist > 40"(M)35"(F)
18.5 or less	Underweight	--	N/A
18.5 - 24.9	Normal	--	N/A
25.0 - 29.9	Overweight	Increased	High
30.0 - 34.9	Obese	High	Very High
35.0 - 39.9	Obese	Very High	Very High
40 or greater	Extremely Obese	Extremely High	Extremely High

FIGURE 2-5
BMI AND WAIST SIZE CALCULATORS

Ideal Candidates for Liposuction

An underlying weight problem may prevent the surgeon from achieving the best results, no matter how great his skill.

To determine if a person is a good candidate for liposuction, the doctor will do a complete physical exam, giving special attention to the area to be treated. The patient's state of mind and psychological health will also be evaluated.

Some individuals are better able to undergo a cosmetic procedure than others. Liposuction is not a cure for obesity, nor is it a cure for emotional problems or trauma. Liposuction simply produces improvement in localized areas of the body.

A person suffering from chronic depression or someone with a distorted body image may not be accepted as a patient. Before considering liposuction, ask yourself these questions:

- Why do I want this surgery now?
- What changes do I expect to take place in my life after the procedure?
- Does my appearance hinder me from participating in certain activities?
- Do I constantly think about my physical appearance?
- On average, how much time in a day do I spend thinking about how I look?
- What body areas do I dislike the most?
- Can I ever be thin enough?
- Am I afraid of getting too fat?

Treatable Areas

The physician must determine a patient's skin elasticity, the ability of tissue to "bounce back" after a liposuction procedure. If a significant amount of skin can be grasped between finger and thumb when pulled away from the body and bounce back, the tissue should tolerate liposuction well.

The most responsive areas are the abdomen, love handles, and thighs. Areas that are a little more difficult to treat — but where good results can still be seen — are the neck, back, hips, and buttocks.

Pre-Existing Conditions

Certain pre-existing conditions (including severe heart or blood pressure problems), presence of infection, and ailments such as diabetes or liver disease may prevent a patient from undergoing liposuction.

Chronic disease or illness can increase the risk of complications, so a prospective patient with significant medical problems should see a family doctor or specialist before cosmetic surgery.

The Effects of Medication

Some medications must be stopped at least two weeks prior to surgery. Your doctor will tell you which medications to continue and those that must be avoided. They include over-the-counter medications like aspirin**, vitamins, and holistic herbs. **CHECK YOUR MEDICATIONS FOR THE PRESENCE OF ASPIRIN OR IBUPROPHEN.

A list of common herbal supplements and the potential problems they can cause are listed in Figure 2-6. Figure 2-7 includes other items to discontinue before surgery.

ECHINECEA	May cause reaction to or reduce the effectiveness of immune-suppressants
EPHEDRA	May disrupt heart rhythm, increase blood pressure, or cause stroke
GARLIC	May increase the risk of internal bleeding
GINKGO BILOBA	May cause the risk of internal bleeding
GINSENG	May increase the risk of bleeding; may cause hypoglycemia
KAVA	May increase the sedative effects of anesthesia
ST. JOHN'S WORT	May inhibit the effects of various surgical medications
VALERIAN ROOT	May increase the effects of anesthesia

FIGURE 2-6
HERBAL SUPPLEMENTS TO DISCONTINUE

ALOE	GINGER	PC-SPES
BILBERRY	GOLDENSEAL	FISH OIL
CAYENNE	LICORICE	VITAMIN E
FLAX OIL	FEVERFEW	MELATONIN
OMEGA 3, 6, 9	YOHIMBE (NATURAL VIAGRA)	DIET PILLS (PRESCRIPTION AND NON-PRESCRIPTION) SUCH AS PHEN-FEN, FASTIN, OR MAHUANG

FIGURE 2-7
DISCONTINUE 2 WEEKS BEFORE SURGERY

Lab Requirements

The minimum lab requirement for outpatient surgical procedures is a complete blood workup (CBC) and urinalysis (UA). A patient over forty may also need an electrocardiogram (EKG).

These tests may seem unnecessary, but liposuction *is* surgery, so thorough medical screening is essential.

All past and present medical conditions should be discussed with your doctor prior to surgery.

A history of stroke, heart valve replacement, or the need for blood-thinning medication may preclude elective surgery such as liposuction.

Recovery

After your procedure, you'll need adequate time away from work and physical activity to relax and start healing. Generally, the more areas treated and the larger the patient, the longer the recovery time.

I usually recommend a minimum of three to four days after a simple procedure, but more extensive surgeries require more recovery time. After resting to allow the body to begin healing, you may return to work and light activities, but nothing strenuous.

There will be some bruising, swelling, and discomfort for a few days. The discomfort is similar to the feeling after a good workout at the gym, not severe pain. If you experience acute pain, contact your surgeon immediately.

Psychological Fitness

A patient should have realistic expectations of improvement, not perfection. The ideal candidate views liposuction as a way to get rid of localized areas of fat, recognizing that it's not going to miraculously change his life.

A prospective patient should make the decision for liposuction based on knowledge about the procedure, and be comfortable with that decision.

Don't be influenced by friends or relatives to have liposuction or *any* cosmetic procedure. Don't assume that surgery will mend a marriage or help you get a better job. Sadly, some patients request multiple procedures, chasing an illusion of perfection. Liposuction alters outward appearance, not problems within.

Patients with Depression

Patients who suffer from chronic depression may experience depression post-op. This can occur within days after surgery and may last for weeks. If you suffer from depression, discuss with your physician how to prevent a post-operative emotional roller coaster.

Choosing a Liposuction Procedure

There's a saying, and rightly so, that 30 is the new 20, 40 is the new 30, 50 is the new 40, and so on. The best candidates for liposuction want to look as good as they feel. Liposuction can help them achieve that goal.

To make an informed decision about the "best man for the job", a patient should thoroughly research surgeons who perform liposuction, and make the selection based on that information.

It's especially helpful to talk to post-surgical patients about their procedures, and the support they received before and after surgery. Their feedback can show the doctor's level of concern for his patients, interaction with his staff, and post-op care.

Previously-treated patients can also help dispel your concerns about the procedure, the level of discomfort you might feel, and how long recovery will take.

Ask your doctor for a list of patients to contact. Prepare the questions you want to ask (examples follow), and select several patients to call.

Questions to Ask Previous Patients

- What procedure did you have?
- How long has it been since the procedure?
- How do you feel about the results?
- Did the doctor listen to your questions and answer them to your satisfaction?
- Is there anything you wish you'd known before the procedure?
- Was the staff friendly and caring, and did they respond to your concerns quickly?
- Would you have the procedure again, knowing what you know now?

Rumors and horror stories about liposuction exist. Most patients understand that those stories have been exaggerated, and are very pleased with the results of their procedures. In fact, many of my patients say that they wish they'd had their procedures sooner.

What to Expect During Recovery

There will be significant drainage on the day of the procedure, and you may feel weak or be mildly disoriented from the medications.

Patients generally experience minimal discomfort; actual pain is unusual. There will be a significant amount of swelling. The incisions will ooze pinkish fluid for a day or two. Slight bruising is also common. These symptoms usually last approximately one week.

You may get up and begin walking the day after surgery, but mustn't return to a full exercise routine for 10-14 days. After approximately 3-6 months, swelling will be minimal, and you should see improved body contours, with barely-visible incision sites.

The Doctor-Patient Relationship

Patients who are well-informed prior to surgery and are proactive post-op have the fastest and easiest recoveries. Apply ice packs to the treated areas, elevate as directed, and use post-operative medications from the *Rapid Recovery®* list.

A good surgeon encourages questions prior to the procedure, and answers all of them to the patient's satisfaction.

The day of your surgery, the doctor should communicate his pre-operative "game plan", and mark all surgical and optional incision sites, as discussed with you. Any final questions can be asked so you'll be completely comfortable with the procedure and confident in the doctor's ability.

When doctor and patient develop a rapport, the medical procedure can be a great experience because with open communication, there will be no surprises…only a new and more youthful you!

3

Choosing a Surgeon Who's Right for You

BEFORE MAKING ANY major decision, you should do as much research as possible. Selecting a physician to perform your cosmetic procedure is one of those major decisions.

A surgeon's credentials are only part of what a patient needs to know. All physicians study extensively and may have years of experience. Most provide satisfactory results in their fields.

But the best experience is gained through hands-on training in the operating room, not from textbook lectures. Consequently, meeting the physician and seeing before-and-after pictures of patients is critical to making an informed choice of a surgeon. Speaking to former patients can also help you evaluate a doctor's skill.

Board Certification

Just because a physician is recently board-certified doesn't automatically mean he's the best-qualified to perform your surgical procedure. Many older physicians didn't initially train in liposuction since it didn't exist when they attended medical school. However, by taking post-graduate courses and performing the procedure consistently, they could excel in the field of liposuction.

Board certification (Plastic, Cosmetic, Dermatologic) indicates a high level of education but shouldn't be the only reason for choosing a doctor. The degree of experience he has is also significant.

Finding the right doctor isn't easy. What used to be called a "bedside manner" is still important. The surgeon should be able to explain medical terms and procedures in language you can understand. He should describe his training and expertise clearly and concisely. A good physician also welcomes any questions you have, and is able to answer them in layman's terms.

Shopping for a doctor may be an unfamiliar concept, but it's very important to help you make an informed decision. You need to find the physician with the right combination of training and experience to fit your needs.

I suggest making appointments with at least three surgeons before seeing the first doctor. You may be satisfied with the first, but even more sold on the last. Don't jump at the first option.

To help make your decision about a surgeon, you'll find a list of questions in Chapter 4 to ask at initial consultations. Frequently-asked questions and answers are included, to help you evaluate the physicians during interviews.

There are some things you'll need to know before your consultations. Confirm that each physician is in good standing with the local medical society, get a copy of his office practice history, and confirm that he has no (or few) malpractice complaints filed against him.

When you meet the doctor, ask what percentage of his surgeries is devoted to liposuction and how often he performs liposuction on a weekly basis. Every patient deserves optimal results. The more a procedure is performed, the better the results.

Don't be afraid to ask questions; it's better to ask them before than after the fact. By being proactive and following the doctor's instructions, a patient can speed recovery and ensure the best outcome after a surgical procedure.

The Procedure: Hospital or Surgery Center?

Some patients assume that medical procedures always take place in a hospital. Not necessarily. While some surgeons prefer ambulatory surgical centers or hospitals (which add to the procedure cost), many plastic surgery and cosmetic procedures are performed on an outpatient basis in an office surgical center.

In the past, to be accredited, hospitals were inspected, reviewed, and approved. That was before office surgical centers existed. Now, surgical centers are used for a variety of outpatient procedures.

It's imperative that the facility is licensed by the state and certified by a recognized accrediting board. That organization also verifies that the surgeon has privileges at a nearby hospital in the event a patient requires transfer to that facility in an emergency.

Administration of Anesthesia

Anesthesia keeps the patient comfortable during and after surgery, and is chosen by the physician based on the type of procedure. The accrediting organization certifies the types of anesthesia that may be administered in the facility, and controls their use.

Your surgeon may be assisted during the procedure by an anesthetist, nurse anesthetist, physician's assistant, or registered nurse to provide sedation and monitor vital signs.

Keeping the patient comfortably sedated is much less invasive than rendering him unconscious.

The extended medical team may consist of circulating nurses, scrub technicians, and other related health professionals. The patient generally sees them just prior to the procedure.

You can request a meeting with the surgical team ahead of time to get a better feel for the medical facility, the staff, and the physician. The way you're treated pre-op is a good measure of the overall operation of the facility.

I recommend touring the surgical facility to gauge its overall cleanliness. If a facility has a less-than-tidy waiting room, wouldn't you suspect a similar lack of cleanliness in the surgical area? Would you choose that facility and risk possible infection or complications? Probably not!

Interviewing Prospective Candidates

After researching physicians, narrow your list to two or three candidates, and schedule consultations with them. Take notes at each interview (see Chapter 4 for sample questions) so you'll remember specific points about each physician. Here are some other things to consider.

Office Environment

Is the medical office pleasant and inviting? Is it orderly and clean? A chaotic lobby area could indicate disorganization in the practice itself.

Is the staff friendly? Do they welcome patients warmly? Sitting in the waiting room allows you to observe the front-office staff as they take phone calls, answer questions, and interact with patients.

Note the time it takes before post-operative patients are seen by the physician. Consider asking them about their experiences with office personnel and the surgeon.

You can expect to be seen for an appointment within a realistic amount of time. Sometimes situations occur that are beyond control, like a procedure that takes longer than scheduled. If your appointment is delayed, the front desk staff should keep you apprised, and be able to estimate how much longer you'll have to wait.

Consultation with the Physician

At your initial consultation, you'll meet with a consultant or patient-care coordinator, but expect to spend a reasonable amount of time with the physician. Ask for brochures about the procedures he performs, and get website addresses you can access from home.

Most cosmetic surgery practices have before-and-after photos for prospective patients to review. These are usually from the best-case scenarios of many surgeries. Keep in mind that the outcomes in those pictures are optimal — or they wouldn't be in the files!

Ask if the before-and-after photos are of the surgeon's actual patients. If not, ask to see pictures of his patients. Run the other way if he says, "No."

Concentrate on pictures of the procedure you're interested in having; it's important that the patients had problems or concerns similar to yours, to know the results you can hope to see.

Ask the consultant all general questions before you see the physician. That way you can better use your time with the doctor, discussing specifics about your procedure. The right surgeon for you is the one who answers your questions to your satisfaction.

Patients are naturally concerned about altering their appearance, and appreciate when a physician takes time to counsel them. Your doctor should offer suggestions to help you achieve your goals.

The Interview

When you meet a physician you're considering for any medical procedure, it's important that you feel heard. A good consultation is a combination of knowledge, communication, and honesty. To help evaluate your interaction with the surgeon, use the following information as a guide.

- Is the doctor willing to do what you desire rather than what *he* may want? Keep in mind, though, that this is an expert who performs the medical procedure you've selected.
- His observations are based on years of experience and he knows what can and can't be achieved.
- Listen to his suggestions, but if he's adamant about adding procedures you haven't requested, reconsider choosing him as your physician.
- Does he understand your motivation?
- Did he offer any alternative procedure that could give the same results?

The interaction between you and the surgeon should allow you to present your goals and give him the opportunity to communicate how he'd produce results. Finally, tell him anything you consider *un*desirable and hope to avoid.

Establishing Effective Communication

During a consultation, be prepared to provide information on current (or previous) medical problems as well as a list of drugs and any holistic supplements you take (even over-the-counter supplements can affect the procedural outcome). Describe your lifestyle and any information that could affect surgery and recovery.

Overall Impression and Evaluation

Compare doctors after your consultations. Even if you're sold on your first consult, keep appointments with the other physicians on your list. Something may convince you that you'd be more comfortable with another physician after all.

Ask for an Estimate

The fees charged for liposuction depend on several factors, including area of the country, specialty, abilities of the surgeon, and reputation.

Get an estimate for a procedure in writing. The quote should give details about costs, inclusions, and exclusions for the entire procedure. A written estimate helps you compare surgeons and what they offer for the amount quoted.

Liposuction costs can vary depending on the area to be treated (and *how many* areas are treated) at once. For example, if treatment of the first liposuction area ranges from $2,000-$4,000, then each additional area might be half of that, or $1,000-$2,000.

"Getting What You Pay for"

Cost is an important factor to consider before having a cosmetic procedure. Variables that can affect cost are the size and weight of the patient, the time and effort needed to perform the surgery, the cost of an anesthesiologist's services, operating room fees, pre-op lab fees, and post-op items (such as compression garments).

Research the surgeons' qualifications prior to having a procedure. The quality of the results should be more important than cost.

Cost, however, shouldn't be the deciding factor when choosing a physician: you should compare experience, surgical results, and ratings from past patients. The most expensive doctor isn't necessarily the best, contrary to what you might think.

Get estimates from several physicians, to determine a reasonable charge for the procedure you've chosen. Well-trained surgeons with extensive experience produce the best results. By specializing in specific procedures, they're more proficient and consistent in the results they achieve.

A Doctor's Safety Record

Always, *always* investigate a medical provider's safety record. Don't forget to do your research in your eagerness to schedule surgery and see results as quickly as possible. Sadly, famous personalities are in the news daily, not for their film achievements but for their surgeries-gone-wrong.

In conclusion, there's no excuse for less-than-optimal patient care. When choosing a physician, look for a medical practice with a near-perfect safety record. Problems can occur during surgical procedures; a surgeon should be able to solve them quickly and efficiently.

4 | Frequently-Asked Questions

IN THIS CHAPTER you'll find questions I'm most often asked when patients come for liposuction consultations. The answers I give help them decide whether or not a procedure will produce the results they desire.

It pays to do your homework. A competent surgeon should be open to answering your questions. After all, you're putting yourself in his hands; you want to be confident they're *capable* hands.

1. How do I choose a surgeon for liposuction?

Physicians who practice cosmetic surgery complete medical school and residency, usually focusing on a surgical specialty: general surgery, otolaryngology (head and neck surgery), dermatology, or plastic surgery.

After receiving board certification, these physicians continue specific post-residency training in cosmetic surgery, through fellowship programs (one-on-one training with an experienced cosmetic surgeon) or by attending cosmetic surgery workshops, seminars, and lectures. Most cosmetic surgeons are members of the American Academy of Cosmetic Surgery.

2. What is the American Academy of Cosmetic Surgery?

The American Academy of Cosmetic Surgery (AACS) is a professional medical society whose members are dedicated to the art of cosmetic surgery. AACS is the largest multi-specialty organization of cosmetic surgeons in the world.

Another resource that provides a good benchmark of a physician's ability is the American Board of Medical Specialties (ABMS).

3. Why should a Cosmetic Surgeon perform these procedures?

Cosmetic surgery is an art. By incorporating techniques from other surgical disciplines, cosmetic surgeons use their knowledge, skill, and experience to perform the procedures safely, with optimal results.

4. Are plastic surgeons more qualified to perform cosmetic procedures?

No. Most doctors only develop cosmetic surgical expertise through post-residency training. Cosmetic surgeons are dedicated to enhancing a patient's appearance using specialized medical techniques.

Cosmetic surgery is practiced by surgeons from a variety of disciplines including board-certified dermatologists, general surgeons, and otolaryngologists, to name a few. All of these disciplines have contributed to the vital growth of cosmetic surgery.

Unlike cosmetic surgery, plastic surgery deals strictly with repair or reconstruction of physical defects. A plastic surgeon doesn't have more cosmetic surgery experience than any other surgeon without post-residency training.

5. Who are the best candidates to undergo liposuction?

Generally speaking, the best prospective patients want to improve — and be more confident in — the appearance they present. It's not age but health and maturity that determine if a patient is a suitable candidate for a cosmetic procedure.

Young, physically-fit people generally get better results following liposuction since their skin is more resilient and heals quickly. But every person is different. In fact, many older patients have excellent skin resiliency and obtain outstanding results.

On the other hand, patients who have lost a significant amount of weight or have poor skin tone aren't good candidates for liposuction. A thorough physical exam including a diagnosis of the patient's skin condition and elasticity must be done prior to any surgical procedure.

6. Will liposuction help me lose weight?

Patients shouldn't expect dramatic weight loss with liposuction. However, because the fat is removed from specific areas for cosmetic reasons, liposuction can produce significant improvement.

Liposuction is body-sculpting performed in localized areas. It will reduce the size of the areas but may not produce weight loss. For every two liters of fat removed, a person can lose roughly 4 pounds.

Larger patients who have significant liposuction of the abdomen, waist, and lower body report a visible reduction in inches as well as a loss of weight. However, remember that liposuction isn't a substitute for a medically-approved weight loss program.

7. Does liposuction produce permanent results?

If a patient doesn't gain an excessive amount of weight, the new silhouette is permanent. It's important to note here that after a liposuction procedure the body will go through the normal changes associated with the aging process (sagging, for example). Nevertheless, the benefits of liposuction will always be apparent.

Be aware that even moderate weight gain after liposuction will cause fat to build in other areas of the body. The body will retain its overall shape, although larger.

8. Can the fat come back after liposuction?

Liposuction removes fat cells permanently; however this doesn't mean that the patient can't gain weight. While the area treated for liposuction has fewer fat cells than before surgery, those that remain can still expand. It's impossible (and undesirable) to remove every fat cell from an area, but most fat deposits can be greatly reduced.

9. Will liposuction help sagging skin?

Sagging skin usually doesn't improve significantly after liposuction. Liposuction improves the shape of the body, not the quality of skin texture. However, the lipolysis laser can tighten the skin's surface, to some degree.

The overall result depends on the initial condition of the skin, which is based on genetics, elasticity, a history of weight loss or gain, and the degree of sun damage. Your physician will be better able to determine the amount of improvement you can expect, based on your individual characteristics.

10. What happens if I gain weight after liposuction?

The results after liposuction will become less noticeable and dramatic when a patient gains weight. A rule of thumb is that a patient should weigh less by the amount of weight of the removed fat after liposuction.

For example, if a 150-pound woman undergoes two liposuction procedures, each to remove 4 pounds of fat (equal to 1 gallon of fat, total), she should try to keep her weight at or below 142 pounds.

Let's say hypothetically that she gains weight six months after liposuction, returning to 150 pounds. The cosmetic results will still be noticeable, but not optimal. If she gains an additional 15 pounds after liposuction, she'd keep the new body shape, but her results would be less than ideal.

11. If I gain weight after liposuction, where does the fat go?

If a patient gains a significant amount (more than 30 pounds) of weight, fat will accumulate in the fat cells that remain.

For example, if a woman gains weight after liposuction of her hips, outer thighs, and abdomen, the fat will be deposited proportionately elsewhere: breasts, face, back, and legs, for example. The number of fat cells in the treated areas has been reduced, so fat cells elsewhere expand.

Also, liposuction doesn't prevent or alter the aging process. It's natural for the size and location of the body's fat deposits to slowly change with age.

12. What can I expect if I get pregnant after liposuction?

Pregnancy doesn't permanently alter the results of liposuction. If a woman has liposuction and subsequently becomes pregnant, gains weight, gives birth then loses the pregnancy weight, her original liposuction improvements will return, just as if she'd never been pregnant.

13. Will liposuction get rid of post-pregnancy fat in my abdomen?

Yes. Liposuction is excellent in improving the abdomen after pregnancy. In fact, for the vast majority of patients, liposuction provides a better and more natural appearance than a tummy tuck. Additionally, scars are minimal after liposuction — the size of a half grain of rice — and recovery is rapid, usually one or two days.

14. Is there a maximum volume of fat that can be removed through liposuction?

In many states, the amount of pure fat considered safe to remove (sometimes up to 6 liters) is controlled by law. The greater the volume of fat removed during a surgical session the greater the risk of serious complications. If a patient has more than 4-5 liters of fat to be removed, the surgeon should split the liposuction into separate procedures or stages.

If 6 liters of fat or more are to be removed, the procedure is considered "Mega-Lipo", and must be performed in a hospital setting. Some surgeons feel more comfortable keeping the volume they remove to under 4 liters, although this is by no means an industry standard.

15. What happens at my initial consultation?

During the initial consultation, the surgeon will assess your physical and emotional health and discuss your goals for the procedure. You'll need to provide complete information about:

- Previous surgical procedures
- Past and present medical conditions
- Medications you are taking, including herbal remedies and nutritional supplements
- Past experience with weight loss and any effect it had on your health
- Allergies

16. What is your policy on confidentiality?

You'll be asked whether or not you'll allow the doctor to use your photographs to show potential patients. You have the right to refuse. Be aware of any talk among the office staff about patients. It's important that you keep your procedure between you and your doctor, not everyone in the waiting room.

17. Where will the procedure be performed?

The type of facility where the procedure will take place is an important factor to consider when choosing a surgeon.

Today, liposuction is seldom performed in a hospital or surgical center. Most surgeons prefer using a certified outpatient facility or a surgical suite, either of which is substantially less expensive for the patient.

18. Who certifies the surgical facility to be used?

Most surgery centers are licensed by the state in which they're located and certified by an accrediting agency or board.

19. Who'll be performing the procedure?

This question may seem unnecessary. But it's important that you confirm the surgeon you've selected will indeed perform the procedure, not a "ghost" surgeon, medical student, or doctor-in-training.

20. What type of anesthesia will be used?

Liposuction procedures can be performed under several types of anesthesia. Your surgeon could use any of these: general sedation, tumescent local anesthesia, conscious ("twilight") sedation, or oral medication sedation.

The surgeon should clearly explain the type of anesthesia to be used for your procedure, who'll be administering it and what, if any, alternative medications could be used. Also ask how the anesthesia will be monitored during the procedure, and by whom.

21. How should I prepare for my procedure?

Two weeks before surgery, you should discontinue taking aspirin and aspirin-containing products and follow any other instructions given to you by the surgeon. Stop taking Vitamin E supplements.

Some prescriptions may need to be temporarily discontinued. Your surgeon may also require medical clearance from your primary doctor or specialist before performing the procedure.

The table in Figure 4-1 lists part of my *Rapid Recovery Method®*, with vitamins and herbal supplements I recommend in preparation for and following a procedure.

I've spent years researching aids to healing, and find this combination of natural remedies to be optimal. Rapid Recovery is what I practice, but not every doctor you interview will share my philosophy. They may advocate using parts of the regimen or none at all.

You'll receive further instructions from your surgeon, so be sure to read and follow them to the letter.

Finally, you'll need someone to drive you to and from the procedure and stay with you for the first night after surgery. You won't be allowed to drive after being sedated.

1 WEEK BEFORE SURGERY	DOSAGE
Vitamin C	3,000 mg daily
Zinc (chelated, if possible)	100 mg daily
Vitamin B-6	100 mg daily
Mephyton (prescription)	3 X daily
Bactroban Ointment (prescription)	Swab inside each nostril 2 X daily for 5 days
1 DAY POST-OPERATIVE	DOSAGE
Papaya Enzyme	1 tab 4 X daily
Arnica Montana	1 tab 4 X daily
Prescription antibiotic	As directed
Prescription pain med	As directed

FIGURE 4-1

RECOMMENDED VITAMINS AND HERBAL SUPPLEMENTS

22. Will there be much pain after surgery?

Because most patients are facing the unknown, it's easy to have exaggerated fears about pain and complications. Let me put your fears to rest: the pain experienced after liposuction is greatly overstated.

For the first day or two, the treated area will be numb from the local anesthesia. Then most patients describe the discomfort as the same way they feel after a vigorous workout at the gym: much less than they had expected. In many cases, there's no pain at all.

23. How much bruising and swelling should I expect after surgery?

Improved liposuction techniques minimize blood loss and bruising — a result of blood under the skin. Bruising and swelling are directly related to the patient's overall health, or medications taken prior to surgery. Excessive bleeding or bruising can also be caused by the surgeon's aggressiveness or lack of technical ability.

At New Image Cosmetic Surgery, I recommend my Rapid Recovery Method before and following my procedures.

This regime combines holistic and traditional medical techniques that expedite healing and recovery. It includes vitamins and prescription medicines and external ultrasound treatments on the target areas.

In conjunction with my pre- and post-op instructions, the Rapid Recovery Method helps minimize bruising and reduce swelling.

24. How long does recovery take, after the procedure?

Depending on what type of liposuction was performed, expect to be up and around in anywhere from a few days to a week. Allow more time for recovery if multiple areas are treated.

The swelling diminishes over the following weeks, with final results seen after several months. Recovery time varies from person to person and technique to technique, but many individuals can have surgery on Friday and go back to work on Monday.

This doesn't mean they're completely back to normal. There will still be some swelling, bruising, and mild discomfort but not enough to interfere with work. The exception to this is any activity that is strenuous or requires substantial exertion. Your doctor will let you know when you can safely return to a normal workout routine.

25. How soon will I see results?

As soon as you're allowed to remove protective bandages and support garments to shower, results will be evident. However, the body takes some time to heal fully.

On the first post-op day, a patient can usually see 60 to 80 percent improvement. For a few weeks there will be post-operative swelling. The rate at which this swelling subsides depends on the surgeon's procedural technique and method for post-operative care.

When the surgeon makes incisions that remain open after surgery (instead of linear incisions closed with stitches), patients can expect to see 90 percent of the ultimate results within four weeks. When the surgeon closes the incisions with stitches, swelling resolves more slowly, usually within eight to twelve weeks. I prefer using the open-incision technique.

Eighty percent of the bruising will be gone within a couple of months. The majority of swelling will be gone in six months, with continued improvement for up to nine months.

26. What if I have complications?

During your pre-operative visit, the surgeon should discuss possible complications. Although problems are few and far between in liposuction procedures, it's important to know how to contact your surgeon as quickly as possible if you suspect a problem, so he can begin treatment immediately.

27. May I see photos of patients with similar problems and procedures?

Examining before-and-after photos helps a patient evaluate the surgeon's skill and attention to detail. Ask how much time elapsed between the pre- and post-op pictures. Six months to a year is reasonable to expect to see the final results.

28. May I talk to your patients about their procedures?

The physician can give you names of former patients to contact for their recommendations. Satisfied patients should be happy to share their experiences with you.

29. What do liposuction charges include?

In surgery centers or in-office operating rooms, the cost quoted is usually all-inclusive. Patients who need additional or more extensive surgery will generally require more treatment. Prices also vary with economic ups and downs.

In hospitals, charges can be broken into five categories:

- The surgeon's fee
- The anesthesiologist's fee (if applicable)
- Hospital charges, including nursing care and operating room
- Medication and miscellaneous surgical supplies
- Any additional charges

Average liposuction costs are discussed in Chapter 6 of this book, in the sections pertaining to those areas to be treated.

The cost of any surgery can vary significantly between surgeons, medical facilities, and regions of the country. Choosing a surgeon with experience and in whom you have confidence should be considered along with cost.

30. Can I finance my procedure?

Most offices offer financing options. When financing a procedure, be sure to study the agreement document and ask for explanation of anything you don't understand, like interest rates, specific terms, and interest-free options.

31. What is your refund policy?

Surgeons have different cancellation and refund policies. Be sure to understand your options prior to surgery; this information should be included on the initial quote sheet.

By asking specific questions, you can evaluate the doctors based on the answers they give. I recommend choosing several of these basic questions to ask the physicians you're considering for your procedure.

5

A History of Liposuction Techniques

MACHINE-ASSISTED LIPOSUCTION WAS developed in Italy in the 1980s, by Dr. Georgio Fischer, to remove localized deposits of fat. The technique was then perfected by Dr. Pierre F. Fournier in Paris, France.

I had the honor of studying under Drs. Fischer and Fournier, and with Dr. Jeffrey Klein, inventor of Tumescent Liposuction. I consider them to be artists in the field of liposuction, and my personal mentors.

Suction-Assisted Liposuction (SAL)

Suction-Assisted Liposuction was the first fat-removal procedure used, and was considered an important breakthrough in its day. In this process, the surgeon moved a cannula back and forth rapidly through fatty tissue, dislodging fat cells which were then suctioned from the body. SAL is now referred to as "dry" liposuction: no fluid was introduced into the body tissue to help flush the cells out. Recovery time was lengthy; while SAL *did* remove fat cells, it also damaged the surrounding tissue, causing extensive bruising.

Tumescent Liposuction

Tumescent Liposuction was developed by Dr. Jeffrey Klein, and is performed under local anesthesia with sedation. The word *tumescent* is derived from Latin, and means "firmly swollen".

In this "wet" procedure, a special saline solution that contains a small amount of epinephrine is pressed *between* the fat cells, not into them. Epinephrine is a natural hormone that constricts blood vessels and reduces bleeding. The water quickly carries the drug that paralyzes nerves and contracts blood vessels in the target tissues.

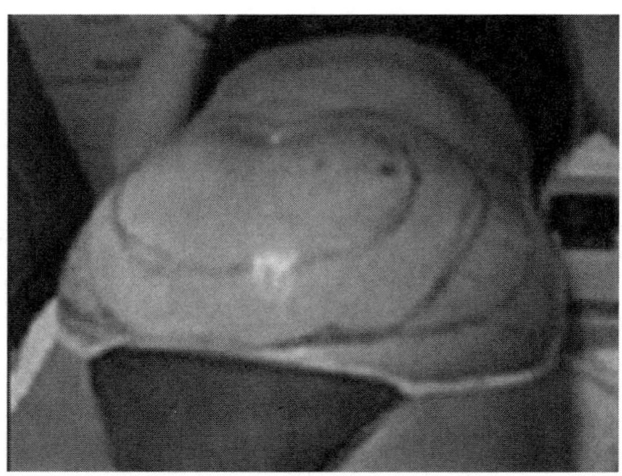

FIGURE 5-1
PATIENT UNDERGOING TUMESCENT LIPOSUCTION

The tumescent fluid "floats" the fat out of the body, limiting blood loss and bruising. This technique minimizes discomfort to the patient, reduces the possibility of complications, and shortens recovery time. Tumescent liposuction has made SAL obsolete, since it provides maximum benefits with minimal downtime for recovery.

Ultrasonic-Assisted Liposuction (UAL)

Ultrasonic-Assisted Liposuction uses a special cannula that transmits high-frequency sound waves into the body. The sound-wave vibration emulsifies fat cells, making it easier for a surgeon to remove the fat.

The ultrasound-transmitting cannula is delicate and precise, and takes specialized skill to use. If used by an inexperienced physician, UAL sound waves can burn the skin.

Power-Assisted Liposuction (PAL)

Some physicians consider *Power-Assisted Liposuction* the ideal procedure to sculpt target areas, since it causes the least amount of trauma to surrounding tissue.

With the introduction of PAL, fewer complications have been seen than with older techniques. PAL employs a mechanized cannula, which the surgeon inserts repeatedly into the fatty tissue. The cannula's vibration disrupts fat cells, causing the fat to detach from surrounding tissue. The fat is flushed out, then suctioned from the body.

External Ultrasonic-Assisted Liposuction (EUAL)

Introduced in the late 1990s, *External Ultrasonic-Assisted Liposuction* uses high-frequency sound waves transmitted through the skin to disrupt and actually liquefy fat cells into the consistency of sour cream. This allows the surgeon to work more superficially, so blood vessels and connective tissue remain intact. EUAL is used to treat larger areas and more fibrous tissues, minimizing blood loss and discomfort.

SmartLipo® — Laser-Assisted Liposuction

SmartLipo is a new form of laser-assisted liposuction. This minimally-invasive technique uses a fiber optic laser to emulsify fat cells. SmartLipo was specifically developed to finely sculpt small areas of resistant fat and tighten the skin.

Under local anesthesia, SmartLipo's minute cannula (holding the laser fiber) is inserted through a tiny incision. As the cannula moves through tissue (shown in Figure 5-2), laser energy permeates the superficial, intermediate, and deep layers of fat.

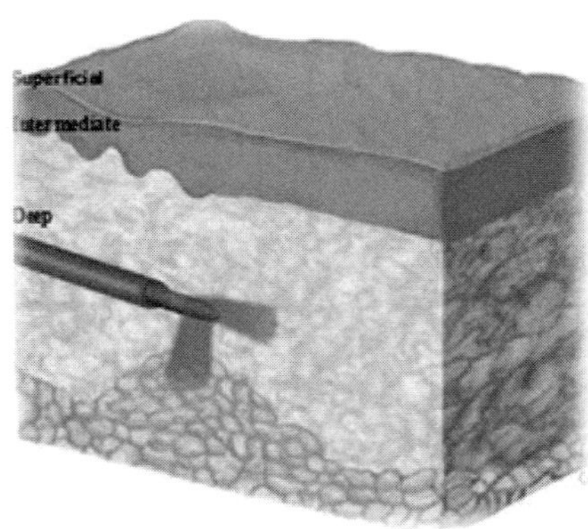

FIGURE 5-2
TISSUE LAYERS, Cynosure Technologies

The procedure is started on a deeper level then gradually moved higher, on a 3-dimensional plane. The cannula is directed horizontally and vertically to ensure symmetrical results.

This process (*laser lipolysis*) ruptures the fat cells, allowing material to be suctioned out. The laser then cauterizes blood vessels, as shown in Figure 5-3, to minimize bleeding and bruising more effectively than earlier techniques.

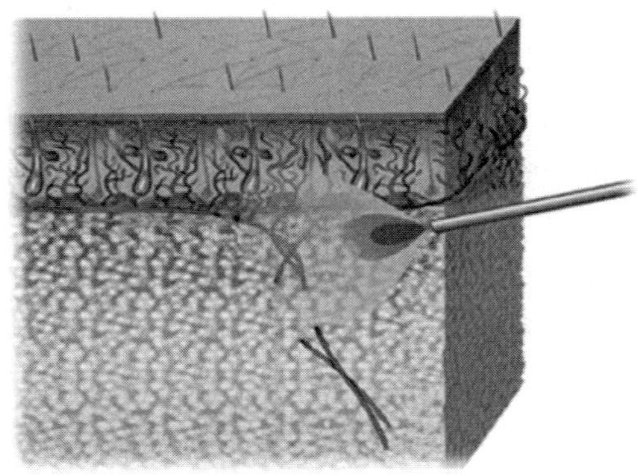

FIGURE 5-3
SMARTLIPO CAUTERIZING BLOOD VESSELS
Cynosure Technologies

Laser lipolysis can treat resistant or difficult areas on the body like scar tissue or naturally dense areas (such as male breast tissue). Its laser wavelength is absorbed by fat which then liquifies, enabling the surgeon to remove it more quickly. Because the cannula is so small, SmartLipo is often used to tighten facial tissue.

The SmartLipo device is shown in Figure 5-4.

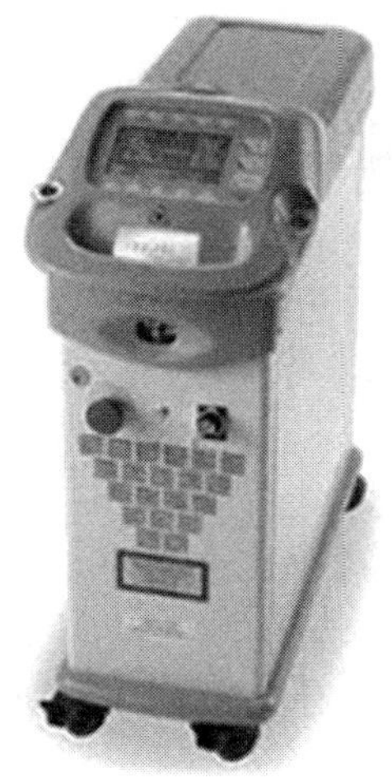

FIGURE 5-4
SMARTLIPO DEVICE
Cynosure Technologies

SlimLipo® — The Name Says It All

In every aspect of life, you need the best tools to get the best results. SlimLipo — _Selective Laser-Induced Melting_ — shown in Figure 5-5, is the newest and best fat reduction treatment on the market today. Other companies make similar machines, but none surpasses SlimLipo. It's revolutionizing the way liposuction is performed.

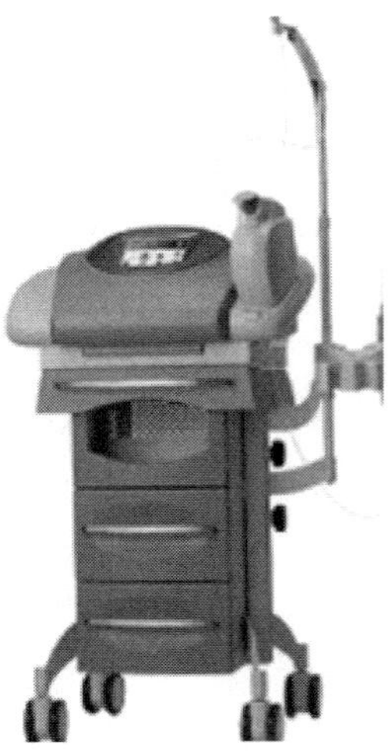

FIGURE 5-5
SLIMLIPO DEVICE
Palomar Technologies

Lasers quickly and selectively heat surrounding tissue to melt fat. The SlimLipo *Stylus Sculptor* causes minimal trauma to the tissues and vessels that surround areas of fat, resulting in less bruising and bleeding. Its unique tip transmits the exact wavelengths needed to melt fat and treat the surrounding tissue. Figure 5-6 shows how SlimLipo melts fat away.

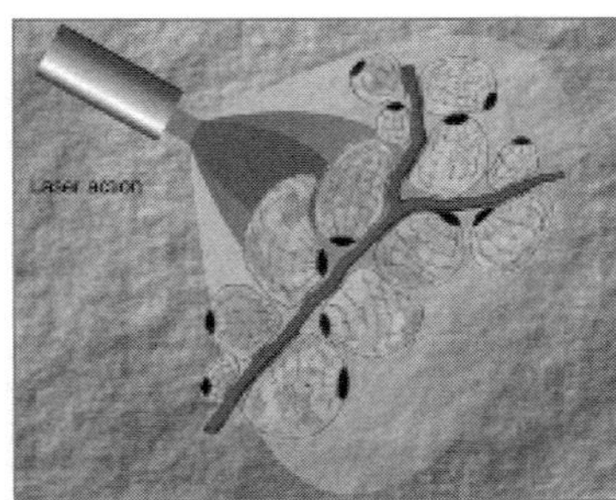

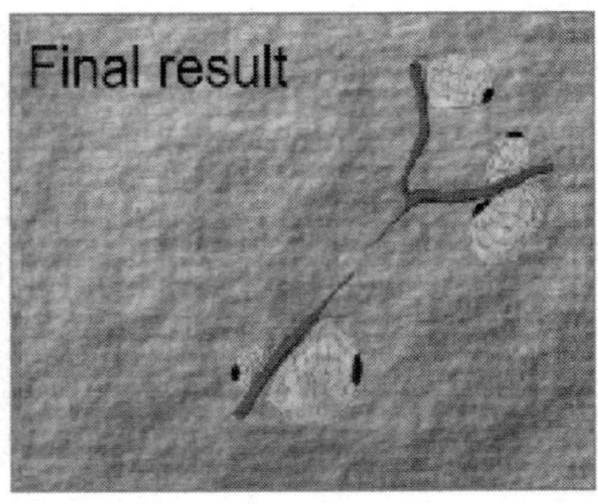

FIGURE 5-6
SLIMLIPO ILLUSTRATION
Cynosure Technologies

Three SlimLipo machines were originally made available for testing, one for me at New Image Cosmetic Surgery, and the other two by surgeons at Harvard Medical and Johns Hopkins University. I personally mentored these physicians in the SlimLipo procedure.

MicroLipo®

In my practice, I use my proprietary technique, *MicroLipo*, which combines these components:

- Tumescent liposuction
- Micro-cannulas
- The *Rapid Recovery Method*®, which I pioneered and developed

At New Image Cosmetic Surgery, I use the newest and most advanced lasers for optimal smoothing and tightening of the skin and underlying tissues. MicroLipo, using *body-jet*, provides excellent results with minimal trauma to the body, which means faster recovery and a quicker return to normal.

body-jet® Liposuction

Liposuction has advanced exponentially with the introduction of *body-jet* (shown in Figure 5-7) technology.

body-jet uses cannula-directed spurts of water to loosen and prepare excess fat cells for removal, much like a power-washer loosens dirt on a driveway.

It was developed in Germany by Human Med AG, and launched in 2004. I was one of the first surgeons to put its technology to work.

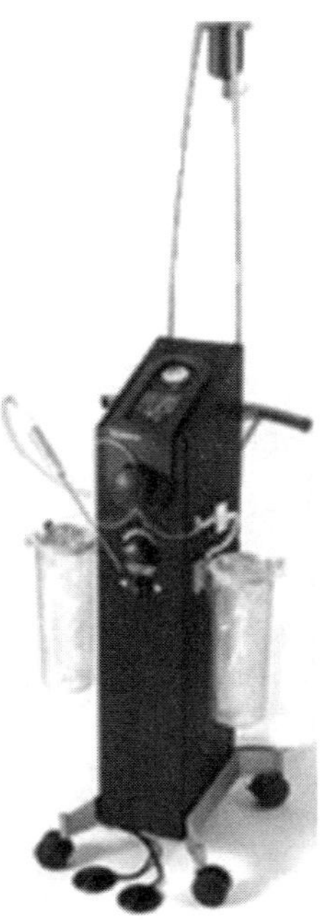

FIGURE 5-7
BODY-JET
Human Med AG, Germany

This minimally-invasive procedure is gentle and effective, producing smoother results than can be achieved with any other liposuction procedures. I'm the first doctor on the West Coast to offer body-jet water-assisted liposuction.

How It Works

Traditional liposuction techniques destroy fat cells, but body-jet loosens the fat without damaging the cell itself. The tip of the cannula anesthetizes tissue, then it rinses out and removes fat while sparing tissue structures, as shown in Figure 5-8.

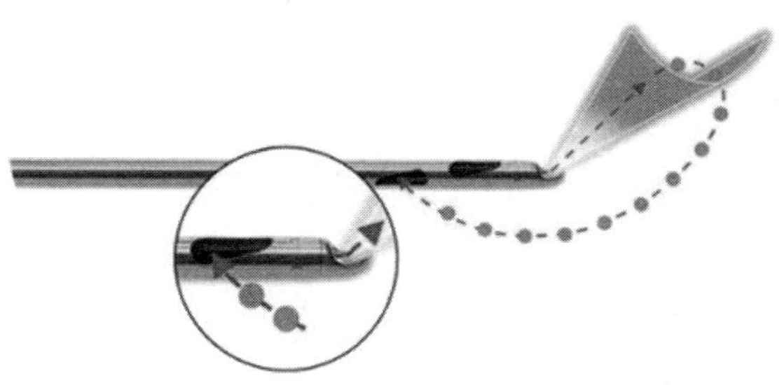

FIGURE 5-8
ANESTHETIC INTRODUCED;
LOOSENED FAT CELLS REMOVED

Its special water solution pushes apart sheets of fat cells at their weakest points, so surrounding structures like blood vessels and connective tissues remain intact.

body-jet uses only minimal tumescent fluid to loosen fat cells – 75 percent less than with standard tumescent liposuction. That means less bruising and swelling, less discomfort, and decreased trauma to tissue. body-jet can be used to treat multiple areas of the body during the same surgical session.

Figure 5-9 shows sketches of the human body, with common liposuction entry ports identified.

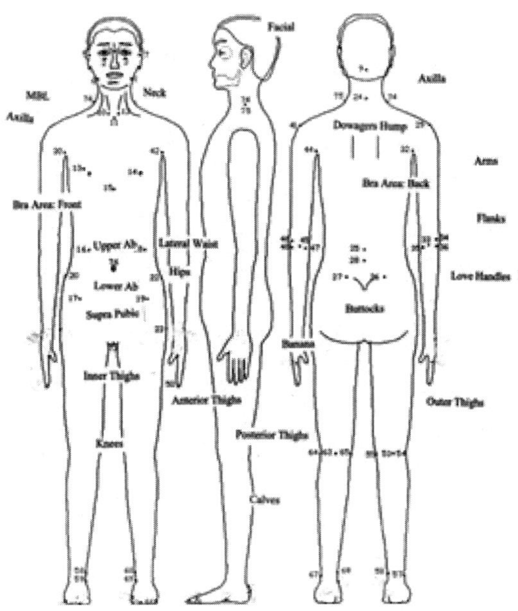

FIGURE 5-9
LIPOSUCTION TREATMENT AREAS AND ENTRY SITES

Fat Transfer

Developing facial wrinkles and creases is a natural part of aging, but excessive frowning, smiling, or squinting can accelerate that process.

Today, a patient's (autologous) fat can be transferred to target areas to fill out lines and refresh facial features. Fat transfer helps define the cheeks and chin, but can also correct facial deformities.

Best of all, since the fat comes from a patient's own body, there's no allergic reaction to the tissue. Finally, harvested fat can be stored for future injections.

Fat transfer is usually done as an outpatient procedure. Both the area from which the fat is taken (usually the thighs, abdomen, or buttocks) and the treatment site are given a local anesthetic.

Using a small needle attached to a syringe, fat is removed from the donor site. The fat is then processed to remove excess fluids, and re-injected under the skin beneath the wrinkle.

This process is repeated until the desired correction has been achieved. This re-injected fat lasts the longest in areas of non-movement, so it's quite effective in correcting sunken cheeks, for example.

Figures 5-10 through 5-14 are photographs of my actual patients, before and after liposuction and fat transfer. Some results are subtle and some are quite dramatic.

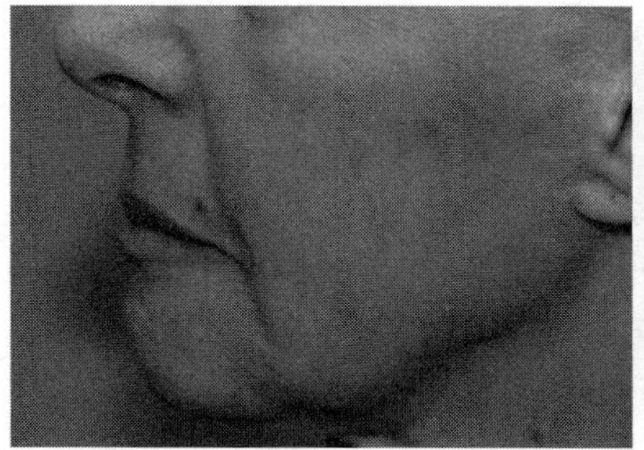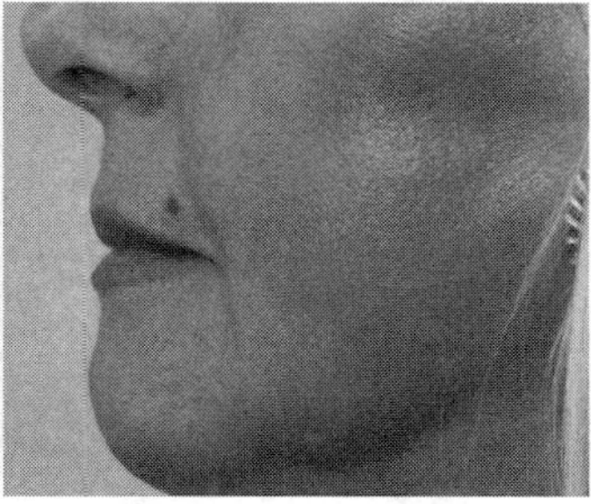

BEFORE   FIGURE 5-10   AFTER

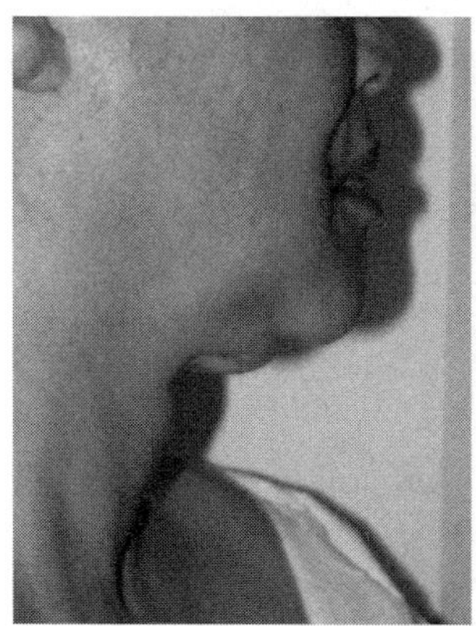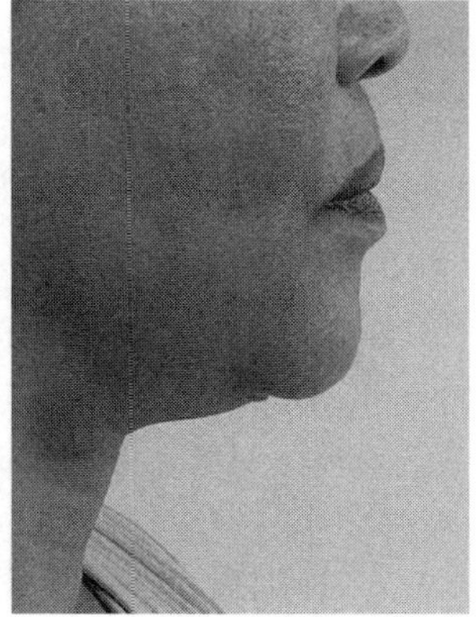

BEFORE   FIGURE 5-11   AFTER

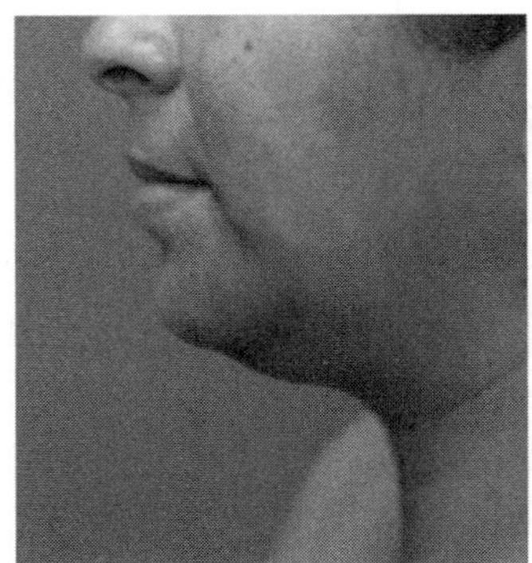 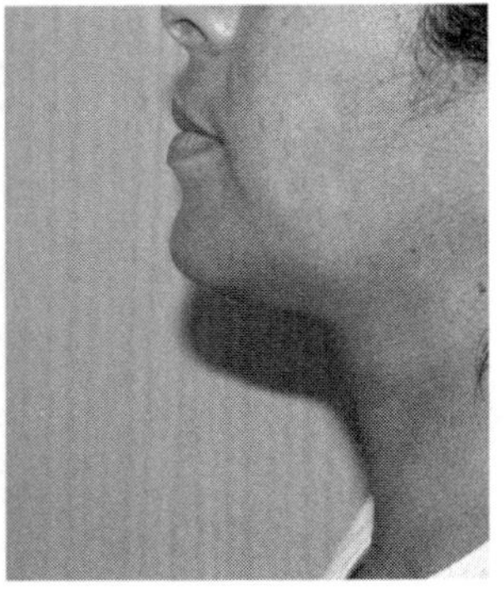

BEFORE   FIGURE 5-12   AFTER

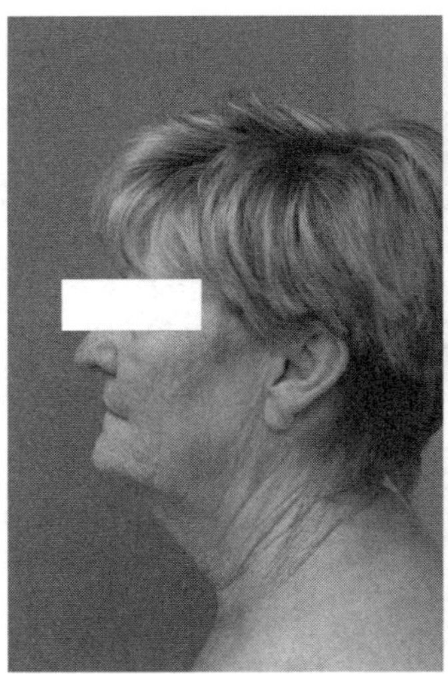 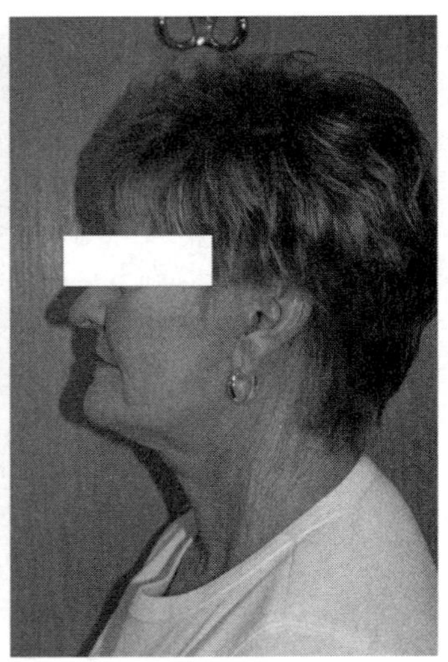

BEFORE   FIGURE 5-13   AFTER

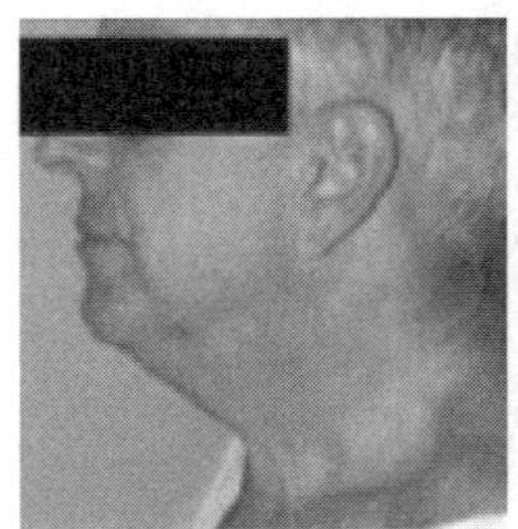 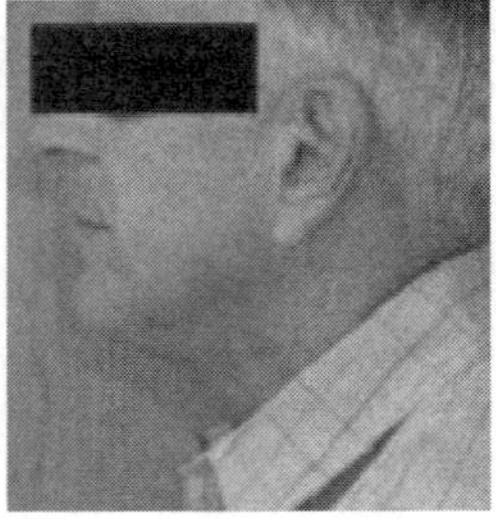

BEFORE   FIGURE 5-14   AFTER

6

Liposuction Procedures

LIPOSUCTION CONTOURS A patient's body by removing pockets of fat from specific areas that are resistant to diet and exercise. Liposuction can produce excellent results in the breasts, upper arms, back, flanks, abdomen, belly, buttocks, thighs, and even the face.

A person contemplating liposuction should research the procedures that will treat their areas of concern, and choose a surgeon based on that specialty.

Following are brief descriptions of common liposuction procedures.

Liposuction of the Breasts

Did you know that liposuction is widely used for breast reduction? Over time, the weight of a heavy breast causes the skin to sag.

Liposuction has been proven to be a less-invasive option for breast reduction for many patients.

Liposuction reduces the volume of fat and can also help elevate the breast. My patient in Figure 6-1 received a two cup-size reduction without losing her breast shape.

MicroLipo breast reduction costs between $2,000 and $5,000, with recovery in four to seven days.

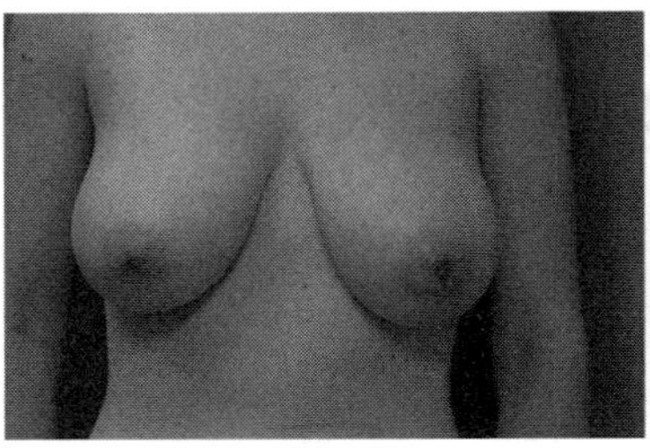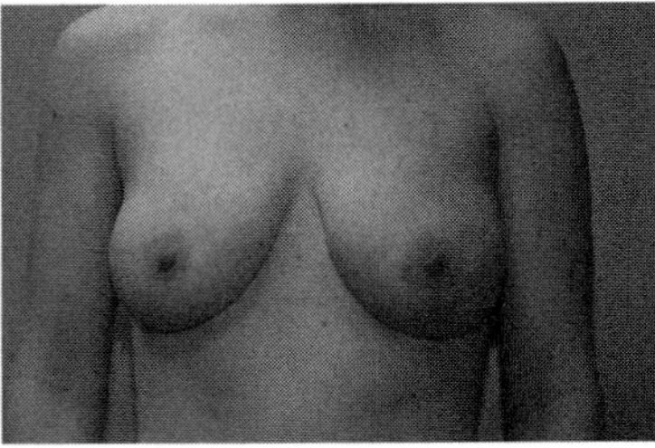

BEFORE   FIGURE 6-1   AFTER
MICROLIPO BREAST REDUCTION
ACTUAL PATIENT

While liposuction can reduce the size of the breast, the overall shape will remain the same. When the breast weight is reduced, skin naturally contracts, elevating the breast slightly.

Liposuction causes minimal post-operative pain, and the patient can usually return to normal activities within a few days.

Contrast that with traditional surgical breast reduction, which involves significant pain after surgery and lengthy downtime. It also results in substantial scarring.

In liposuction, incisions (called *adits*) of less than one mm are made, through which tumescent local anesthesia is infused, followed by insertion of a microcannula to remove fat.

The adits are left open after surgery to enable post-operative drainage, helping reduce swelling and bruising. The incisions are so small that, when healed, the scars are almost invisible.

In breast liposuction, 2 adits are made in each breast. Again, by using tiny incisions, there are no large scars to heal, meaning a faster and virtually pain-free recovery.

Breast reduction using liposuction enables the surgeon to remove up to 50 percent of the breast's volume with minimal risk of complication, and promises a more rapid recovery than with a traditional breast reduction.

Is Breast Liposuction Right for You?

Some women are better candidates for breast liposuction than others. Those with a larger ratio of breast fat to tissue have better results; post-menopausal women fall into this category more often than younger women. In Figure 6-2 you can see the amazing improvement in my patient's profile.

Women who are overweight (not obese) can also expect to see dramatic results from breast liposuction. Prior to the procedure, a mammogram will be performed to determine the amount of fat in a patient's breasts.

It's unrealistic to expect perfect breasts after liposuction. Unfortunately, modern surgical procedures have yet to create a perfect breast.

Liposculpture produces a smaller version of the same breast. Overall shape won't change. But liposuction removes fat, causing the tissue to contract (raising the breast and nipple), for a more "perky" breast.

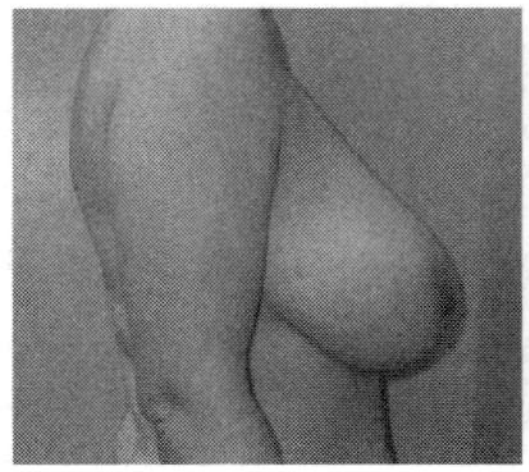 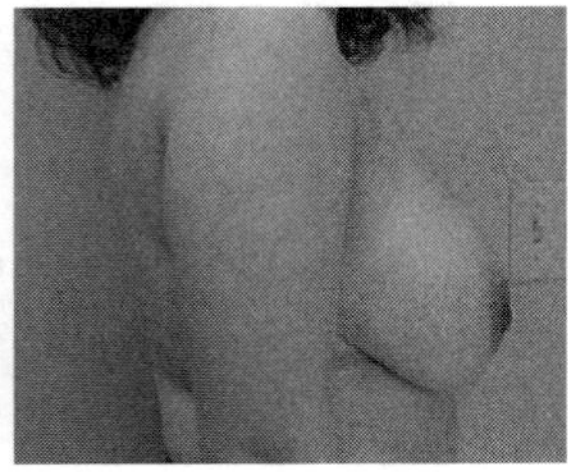

BEFORE   FIGURE 6-2   AFTER
BREASTS WERE REDUCED FROM SIZE F TO SIZE D CUP
WITHOUT REMOVING EXCESS SKIN,
ACTUAL 40-YEAR-OLD PATIENT

Women who have large, pendulous breasts that contain little fat may have skin stretched so taut that it can't physically retract when tissue is removed. Unfortunately, they won't get the same results as others might, but there *will* be noticeable improvement after liposuction.

Women with *gigantomastia* (a condition resulting in excessively large breasts) also benefit from breast liposuction. As mentioned, 50 percent of breast fat can be safely removed, so liposuction is ideal for women with this condition. Although these women will still have very large breasts, they can avoid the scarring caused by traditional breast lift procedures.

Women of child-bearing age frequently ask if they'll still be able to breastfeed after liposuction. In most cases they can. Liposuction performed by a skilled surgeon should cause little damage to the milk ducts, since most of the breast tissue is left intact.

Prior to menopause, breasts have more glandular tissue than fat, which makes the fat more difficult to remove. Post-menopause, breast liposuction is relatively straightforward, since there's a greater amount of fat present in the breasts.

What to Expect After Breast Liposuction

After breast liposuction, patients experience a gradual decrease in post-operative swelling. The use of compression garments can speed the process. It's common to notice "lumpiness" in the breasts for several weeks after surgery. These lumps are a normal part of the healing process.

My Rapid Recovery Method® helps decrease swelling and bruising, enabling the patient to return to normal activities more quickly. Many patients can have breast liposuction on Friday, and return to work on Monday, wearing a compression garment for a few days. They can get back into a light exercise program within a week.

Liposuction of the Upper Arm

Upper-arm liposuction contours and shapes the arms so that they're in proportion with the rest of the body. Fat pads in front of and behind the armpit are sometimes included when performing the upper arm liposuction procedure.

The cost of upper-arm liposuction varies from $2,000 to $4,000, and recovery time is between two and four days.

Liposuction and sculpture of the arms is performed almost exclusively on women. For most, the goal of upper-arm liposuction is to feel lean, defined, and more attractive.

For upper-arm liposuction to be effective, skin should have good elasticity. The skin should contract smoothly and evenly over the area after a moderate amount of fat is removed, as seen in Figure 6-3.

The upper arm area usually heals quickly, and while many surgeons aren't comfortable working in those areas, a surgeon experienced in treating the upper arms can achieve outstanding results.

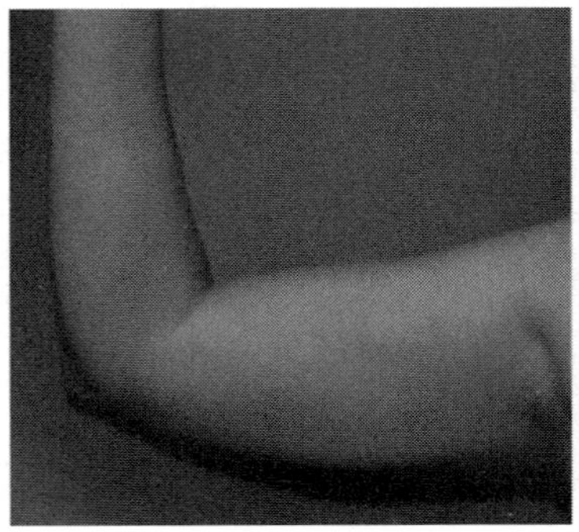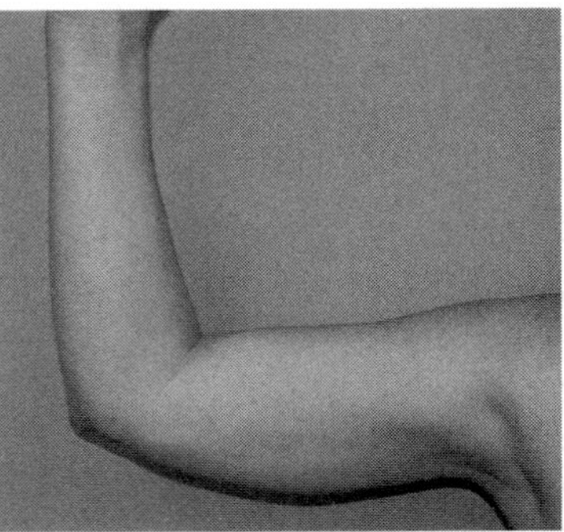

BEFORE   FIGURE 6-3   AFTER
LIPOSUCTION OF UPPER ARM
ACTUAL 40-YEAR-OLD PATIENT

A surgeon should never try to remove the most fat possible. An arm that is disproportionately small is no better than one that's large. Look at it this way: skinny arms on an otherwise buxom woman would look ridiculous.

In the past, the only way to make the arm smaller was to make an incision from the armpit to the elbow to allow the physician to remove fat. The excess skin also had to be excised, the entire length of the upper arm.

This procedure left ugly scars, so the surgery was only performed on previously obese individuals who'd lost a great deal of weight.

In liposuction, small incisions made for the cannula to be inserted are tiny, leaving virtually invisible scars. Excision of skin isn't needed, so there's no scarring from armpit to elbow. In fact, no scars can be seen at all in the patient shown in Figure 6-4.

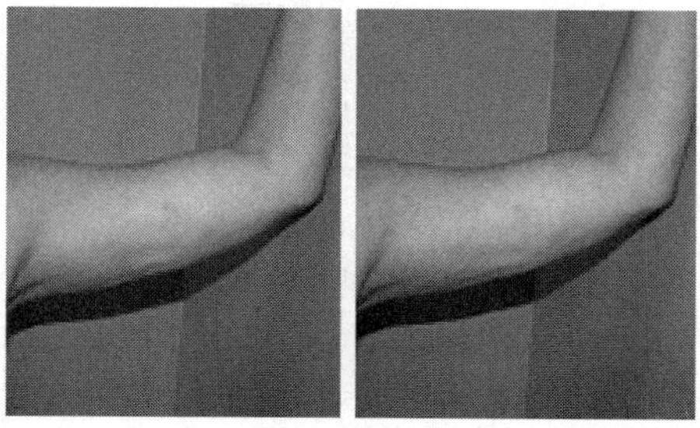

BEFORE   FIGURE 6-4   AFTER
LIPOSCULPTURE OF THE UPPER ARMS
ACTUAL 30-YEAR-OLD PATIENT

The young woman in Figure 6-5 also benefited from minimal liposuction of her upper arms.

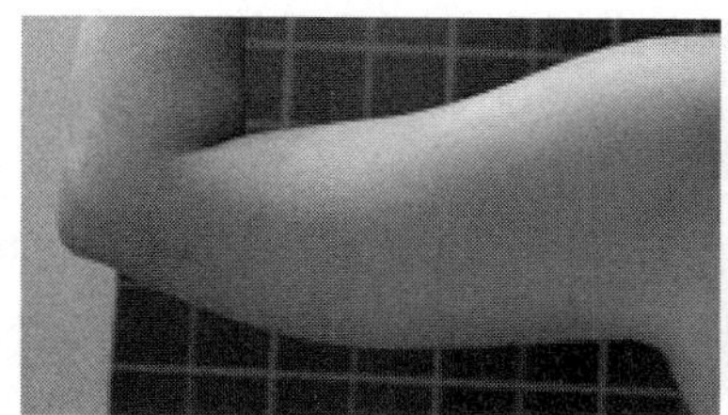
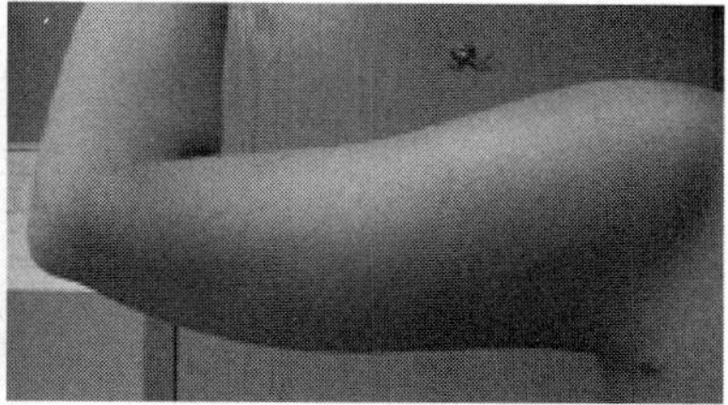

BEFORE   FIGURE 6-5   AFTER
LIPOSCULPTURE OF THE UPPER ARMS
ACTUAL PATIENT

Liposuction is extremely effective for the arms because the fat is removed around the entire circumference of the upper arm. This allows the skin to regain its elasticity evenly.

What to Expect after Upper Arm Liposuction

Moderate compression is needed after liposuction of the arms, and recovery is rapid. Most patients see noticeable improvement within a few days of the procedure.

Some patients experience mild swelling, but can return to normal activity within a few days. In just months, the upper arm will be completely healed, with nearly invisible incision scars.

After successful liposuction surgery, the patient can wear short-sleeved and sleeveless clothing without being embarrassed by flabby, shapeless arms.

Liposuction of the Upper Back and Flanks

Liposuction of the sides and back is typically requested by women, but can be performed on men, as well. Areas of localized fat in the upper back (dorsal) region respond well to liposuction procedures.

The area most bothersome for women is at the bra line. Some women are genetically predisposed to fat accumulation in this area, but obesity also causes fat to settle in the back. Liposuction in this area can give exciting results, when performed by an experienced surgeon.

Liposuction of the back can be more challenging than in other areas because of the fibrous nature of dorsal fat. Overly-aggressive liposuction can cause permanent scarring or discoloration.

Another problem is that the fat isn't concentrated in one area — it's a thick continuous layer, the whole length of the back. Using longer cannulas during the procedure produces the best results, as Figure 6-6 shows.

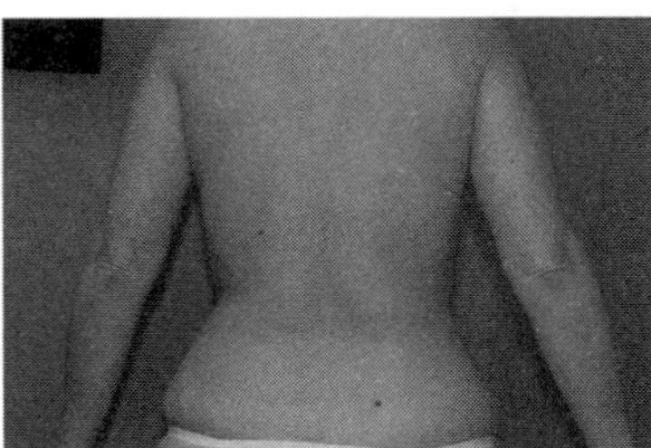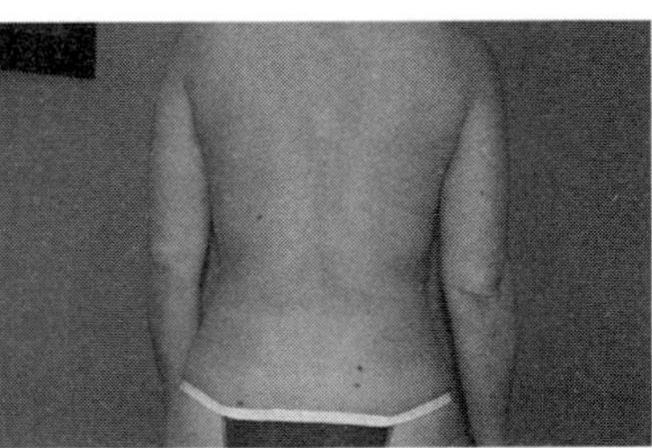

BEFORE   FIGURE 6-6   AFTER
ACTUAL PATIENT

Another area that responds well to liposuction is the cervico-dorsal area in the upper back, below the neck (often called a Buffalo Hump or Dowager's Hump).

Fat accumulates there when an individual gains weight. Patients who undergo this surgery are elated by the great results that can be achieved.

Moving down the back of the body, the next area prone to problem fat is the posterior waist, sometimes overlooked by a surgeon when performing liposuction of the hips. Make sure the surgeon you choose for this procedure will treat that area, too.

Flanks are the areas along the sides of the body between the underarms and the hips. It's common to have fat deposits from just below the underarm down to the waist. You probably know these areas by their more descriptive name: "love handles".

In women, the flanks have more fibrous type of fat, so the surgeon must work very carefully when performing liposuction there. But the results are worth the extra time it takes, giving new shape to the patient's waist. Figures 6-7 and 6-8 show vast improvement in these areas.

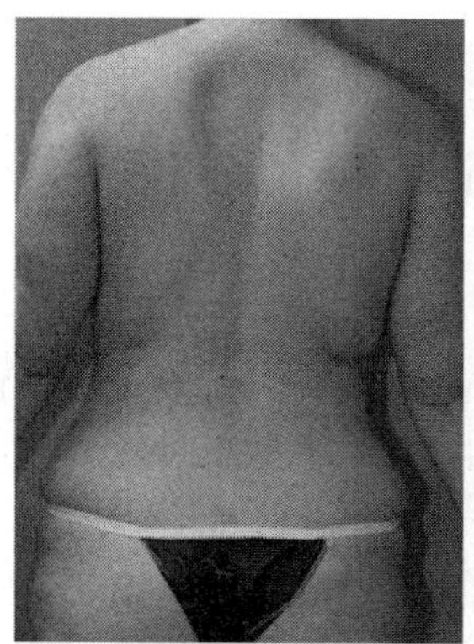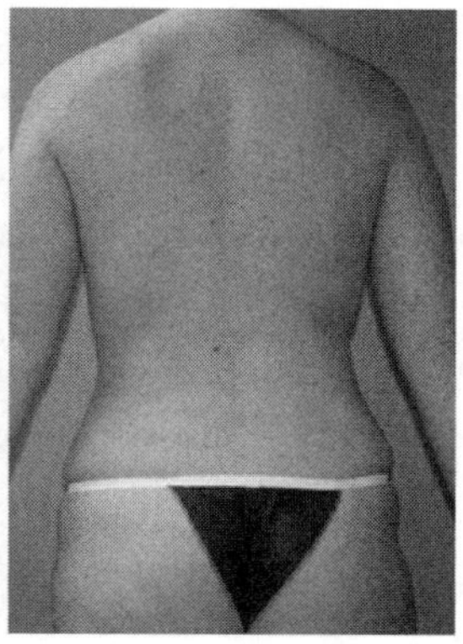

BEFORE   FIGURE 6-7   AFTER
SMARTLIPO OF LOVE HANDLES AND FLANKS
ACTUAL PATIENT

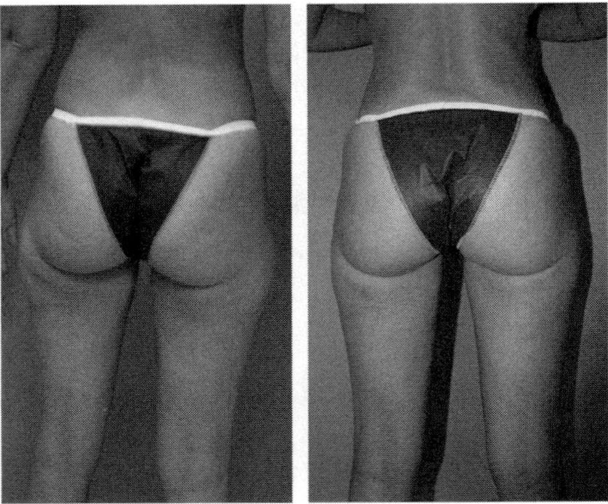

BEFORE   FIGURE 6-8   AFTER
ACTUAL PATIENT

The cost of these procedures varies from $2,000 to $4,000, with recovery within two to four days.

Liposuction of Abdomen and Belly

The abdomen and stomach respond well to liposuction. Both men and women get superior results from the procedure, which varies in cost from $2,000 to $4,000. Recovery time is usually 3 to 5 days.

Abdominal fat can be found in either or both of two tissue layers: subcutaneous and intra-abdominal. The physician must determine which type of fat he's dealing with in the abdomen to know how it will respond to liposuction.

Subcutaneous fat lies between the abdominal wall and the top layers of skin. Fat here responds very well to liposuction.

Intra-abdominal fat is located within the abdominal cavity itself, resting on the intestines. This fat can't be removed by liposuction.

Successful abdominal liposuction depends on the amount and location of abdominal fat, as well as age and sex, whether the patient has had children, and any history of weight gain or loss. Following are some of my patients' before and after photos.

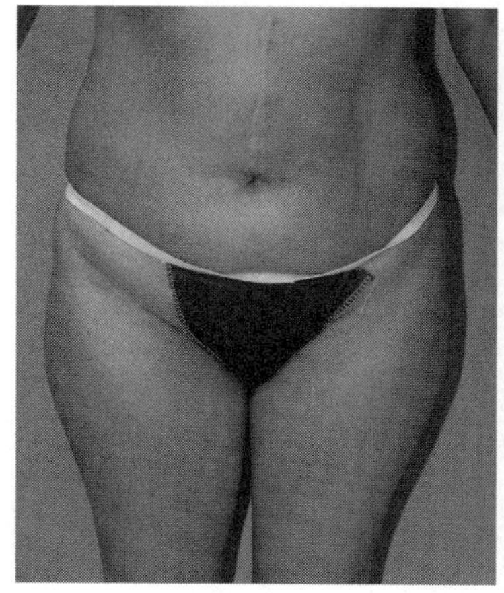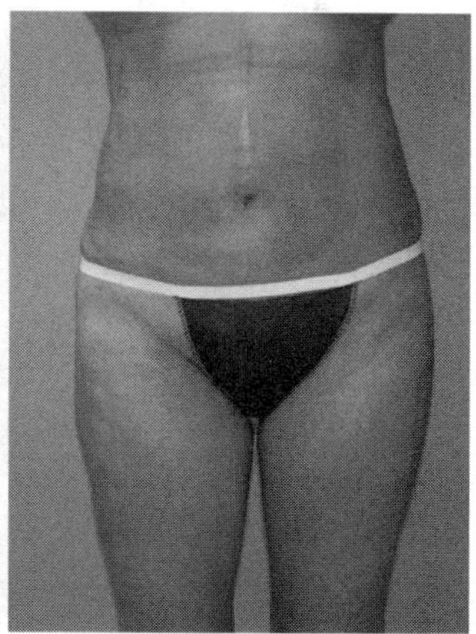

BEFORE   FIGURE 6-9   AFTER
LIPOSUCTION OF HIPS, ABDOMEN, BELLY, AND THIGHS

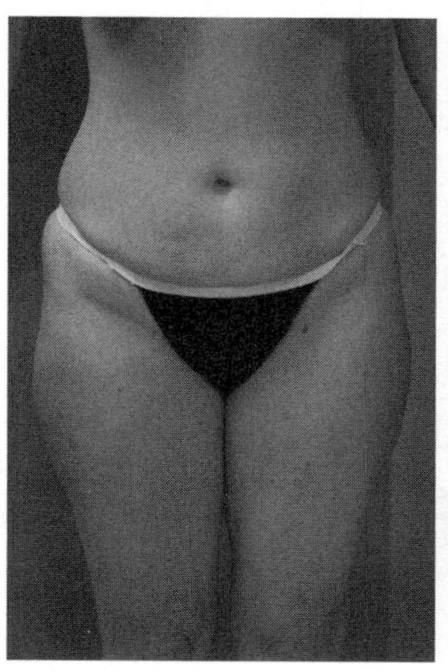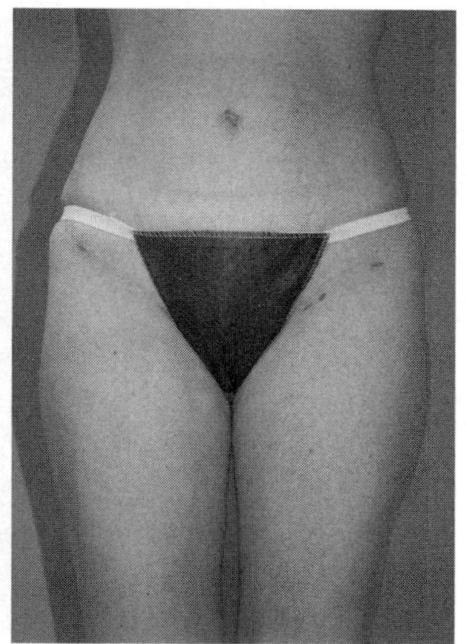

BEFORE   FIGURE 6-10   AFTER
LIPOSUCTION OF HIPS, ABDOMEN, BELLY, AND THIGHS

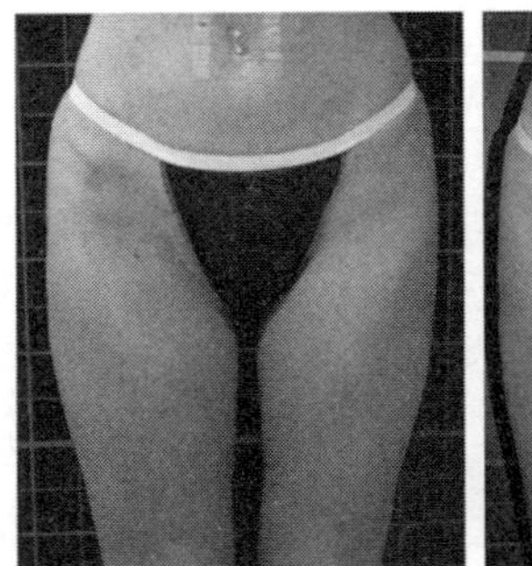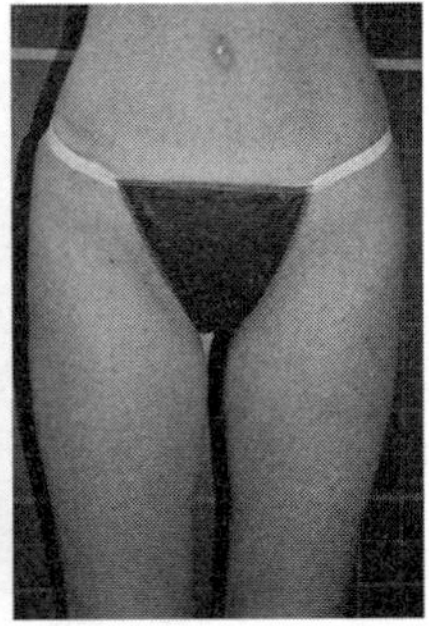

BEFORE   FIGURE 6-11   AFTER
LIPOSUCTION OF HIPS AND ABDOMEN

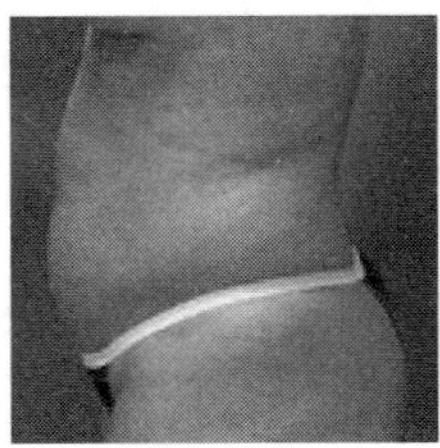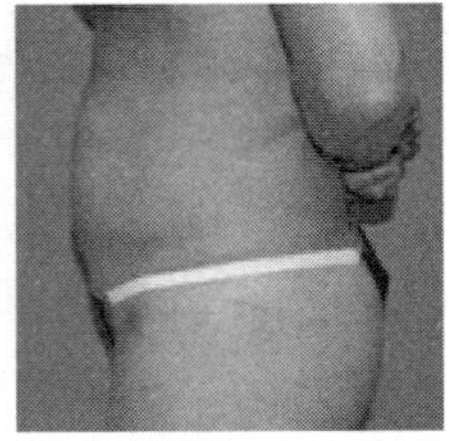

BEFORE   FIGURE 6-12   AFTER
LIPOSUCTION OF THE ABDOMEN

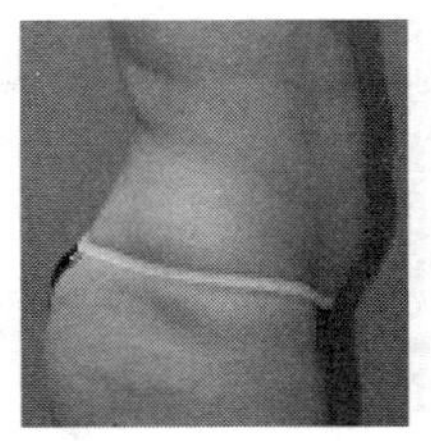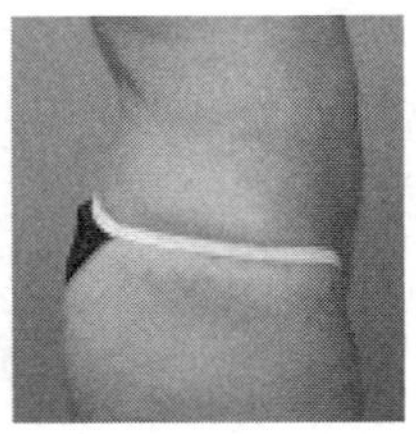

BEFORE   FIGURE 6-13   AFTER
LIPOSUCTION OF THE ABDOMEN

Pregnancy stretches the abdominal muscles, causing the lower abdomen to bulge. How well the abdominal wall muscles retract determines how flat the abdomen will be after liposuction. The vast majority of post-pregnant women who have liposuction don't need tummy tucks after having children.

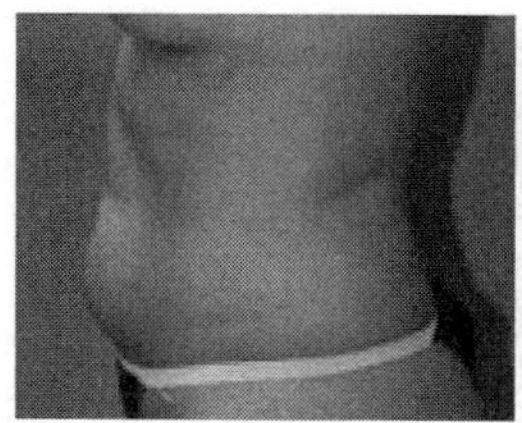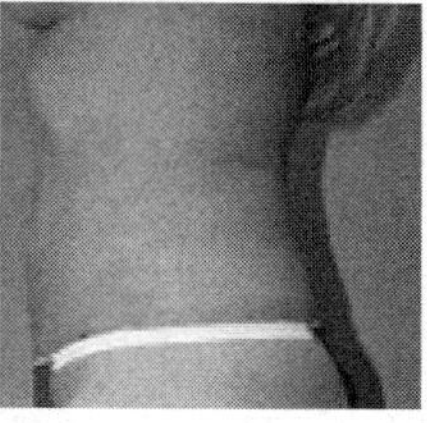

BEFORE   FIGURE 6-14   AFTER
LIPOSUCTION OF THE ABDOMEN, POST-PREGNANCY
ACTUAL PATIENT

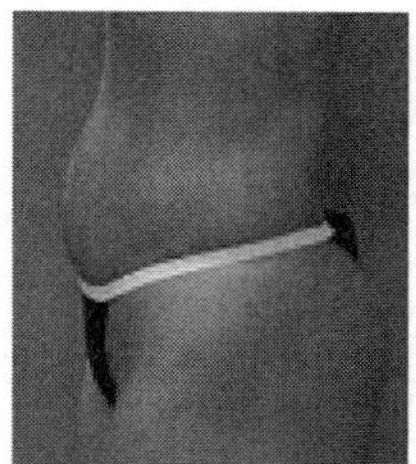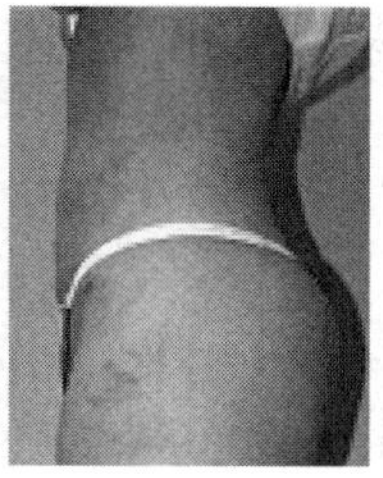

BEFORE   FIGURE 6-15   AFTER
LIPOSUCTION OF THE ABDOMEN, POST-PREGNANCY
ACTUAL PATIENT

A woman who's had a Cesarean section or a hysterectomy made through an abdominal incision can develop a pocket of fat just above the incision. Liposuction can quickly and easily remove this unwanted fat.

Some patients think the only way to get rid of a pendulous abdomen is with a traditional tummy tuck. That invasive procedure leaves the patient with extensive scarring, and carries the risk of infection at the incision site, and can cause blood clots in the lungs. Tummy tucks are also much more expensive than liposuction.

Liposuction is extremely effective in the abdominal area and can produce wonderful results.

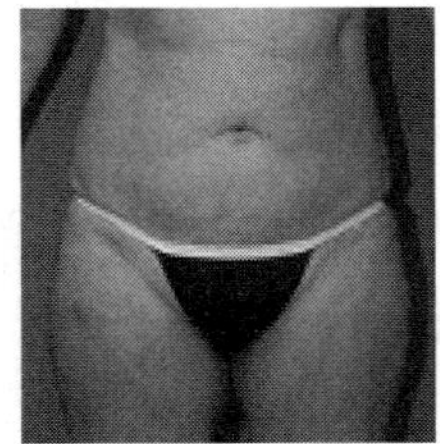 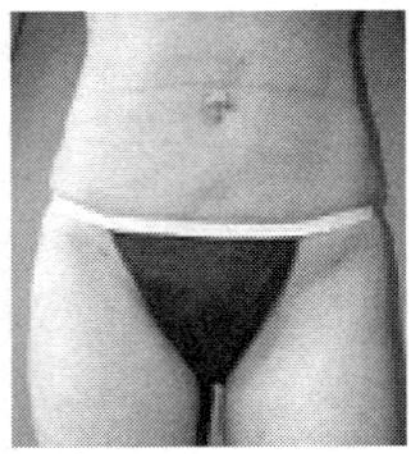

BEFORE   FIGURE 6-16   AFTER
LIPOSUCTION OF ABDOMEN AND THIGHS
ACTUAL PATIENT

The skin of the upper abdomen may be slack after liposuction, especially in older patients whose skin elasticity has decreased. Lower abdominal skin isn't as prone to laxity.

What to Expect After Abdominal Liposuction

Post-operatively, patients who have abdominal liposuction usually describe the pain they experience as minor, treatable with over-the-counter pain relievers. The use of small incisions, tiny cannulas, and local anesthesia means less post-operative pain overall.

If incisions are closed with sutures, the tumescent fluid used in the liposuction procedure can become trapped under the skin, causing prolonged swelling, soreness, and pain. As I mentioned previously, if liposuction incisions are allowed to remain open for a couple of days, fluid can drain, helping decrease pain. The incisions close naturally in a matter of days. A certain amount of swelling, firmness, and lumpiness is normal, subsiding in about twelve weeks.

Results can be seen in a few days, about the time the drainage stops. The area will continue to improve as the swelling goes down.

Figures 6-17 through 6-20 are more abdominal liposuction *before and after* photos of actual post-pregnancy patients.

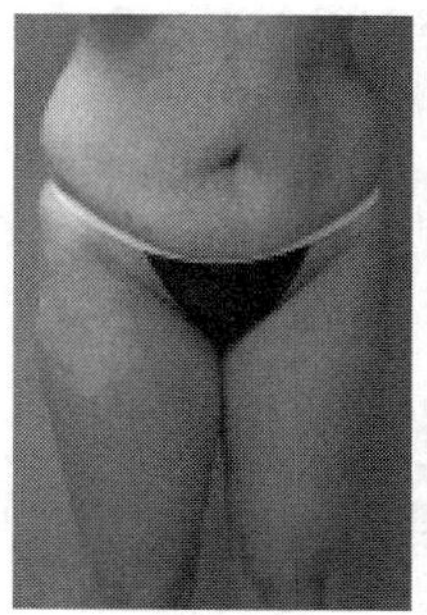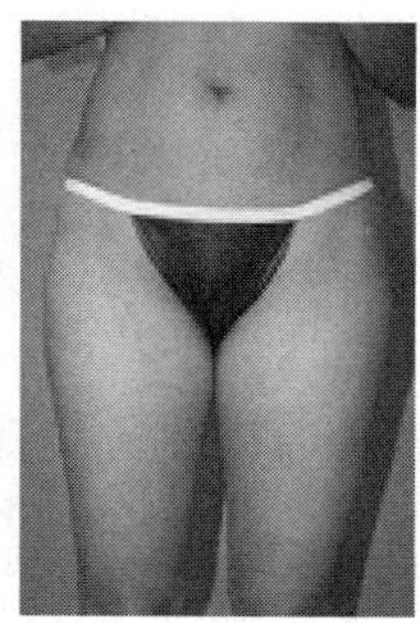

BEFORE   FIGURE 6-17   AFTER
ACTUAL PATIENT

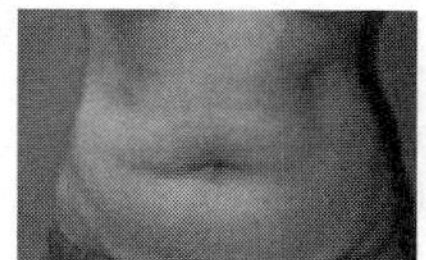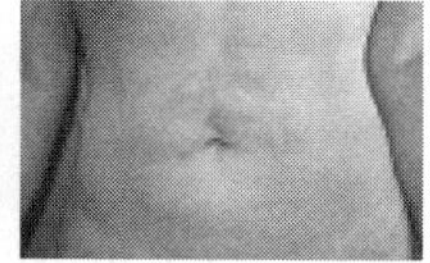

BEFORE   FIGURE 6-18   AFTER
ACTUAL PATIENT

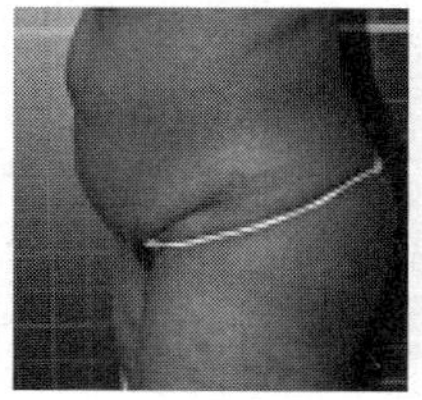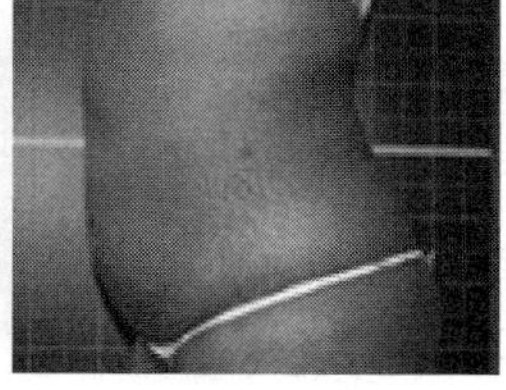

BEFORE   FIGURE 6-19   AFTER
ACTUAL PATIENT

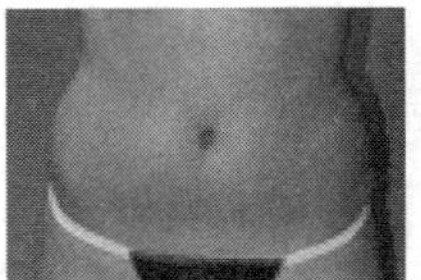 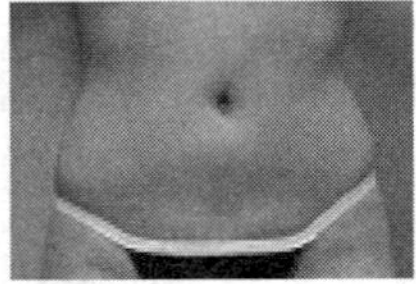

BEFORE   FIGURE 6-20   AFTER
ACTUAL PATIENT

Liposuction of the Buttocks

Buttocks are not only part of the body's symmetry; they also function as the soft cushions that we sit on. When considering liposuction of the buttocks, it's important to remember that maintaining shape is more important than reducing overall size.

Removing too much fatty tissue can result in asymmetrical, lumpy, sagging buttocks. As a rule, no more than 40 percent of buttock fat should be removed by liposuction.

The shape of the buttocks is formed by subcutaneous fat. This area of the body should be treated carefully since the buttocks provide protection to the hipbones and spine when sitting on a hard surface. Tumescent liposuction can beautifully curve buttocks, improving their size and shape.

Liposuction won't noticeably lift the buttocks. Fatty tissue removed evenly from the buttocks can reduce their overall weight, causing the skin to retract, giving the appearance of a slight lift. However, if the skin has lost elasticity, there's not much chance of elevation.

My patient shown in Figure 6-21 was elated with the results that liposuction gave her. The cost of these procedures ranges from $2,000 to $4,000, with three to five days to recover.

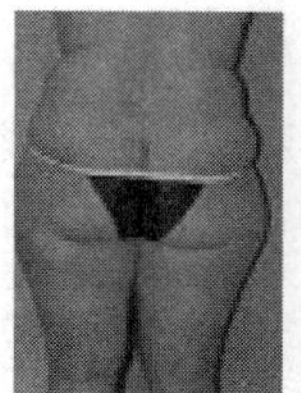 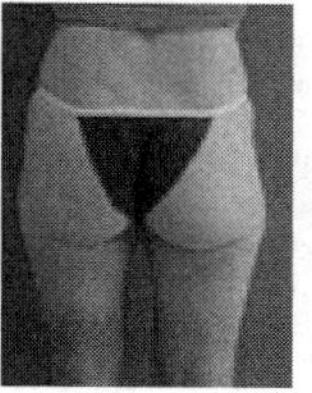

BEFORE   FIGURE 6-21   AFTER
ACTUAL PATIENT

Overly-aggressive liposuction can result in sagging and surgical irregularities of the skin. The surgeon shouldn't remove too much fat but just enough to produce a smooth, natural curve.

Liposuction of the buttocks should be done in the shape of a donut, to uniformly reduce size and bulk, smooth the area, and avoid removing too much fat. Micro-cannulas inserted through tiny incisions leave virtually invisible scars.

The next *before and after* photographs are dramatic examples of what I've achieved using specific liposuction methods on the buttocks (and thighs, in some cases). You'll see a variety of body types and degrees of change. Find a patient whose body structure is similar to yours, and imagine the transformation you could see in your *own* body.

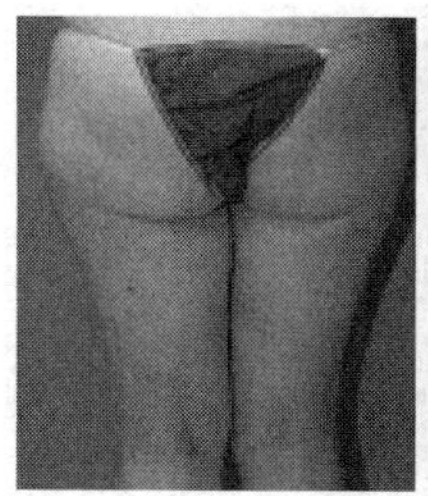 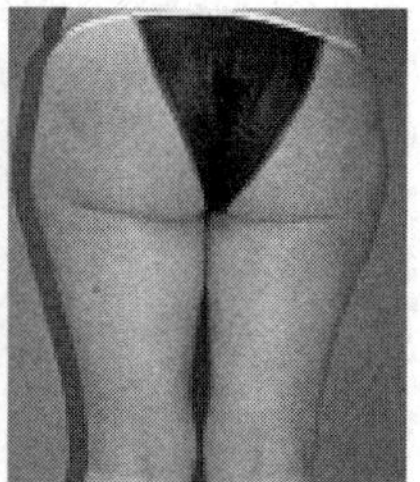

BEFORE   FIGURE 6-22   AFTER
LIPOSUCTION OF BUTTOCKS, FLANKS, AND THIGHS
ACTUAL PATIENT

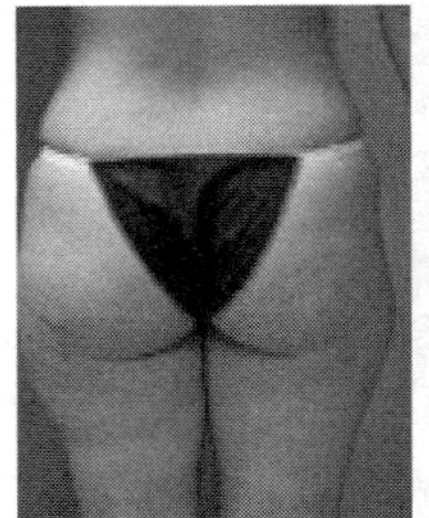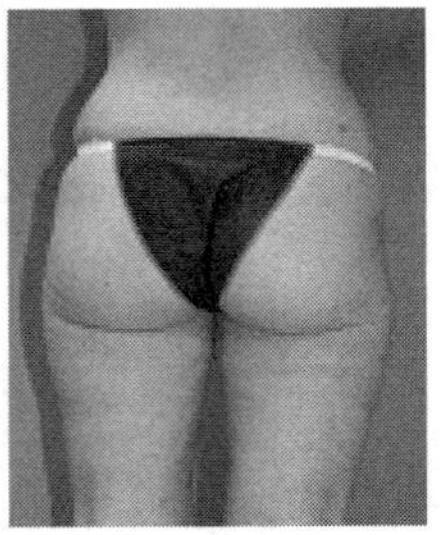

BEFORE   FIGURE 6-23   AFTER
ACTUAL PATIENT

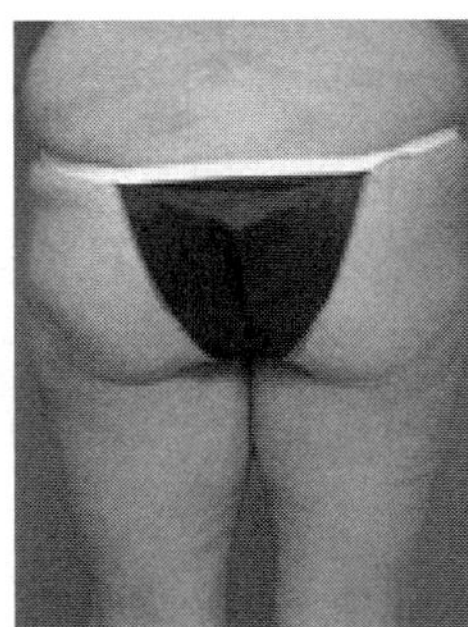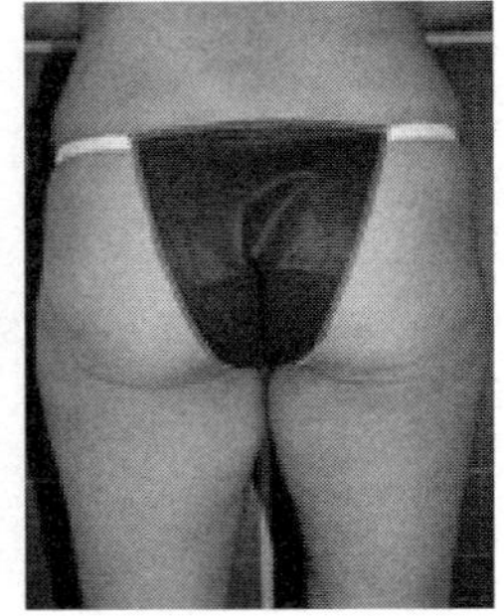

BEFORE   FIGURE 6-24   AFTER
ACTUAL PATIENT

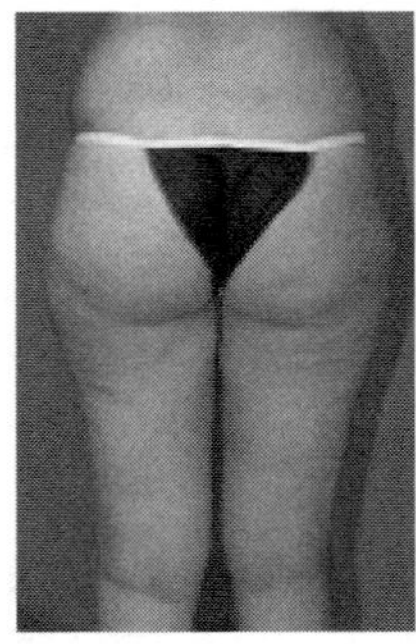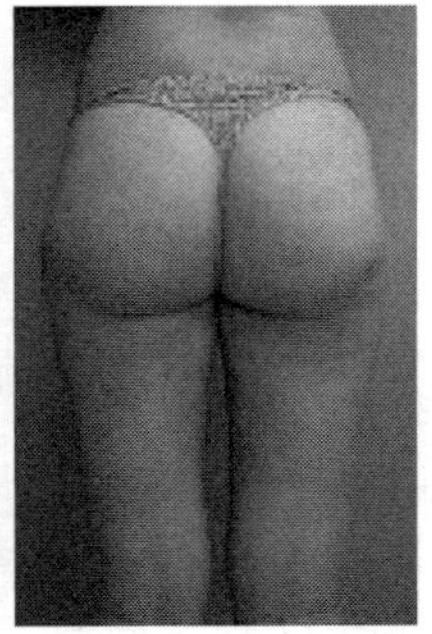

BEFORE   FIGURE 6-25   AFTER
ACTUAL PATIENT

Liposuction of the Hips and Thighs

The fat that women get on their hips and thighs is largely determined by heredity. Unfortunately, those areas are also resistant to dieting and exercise. But liposuction can correct the tendency to store fat there.

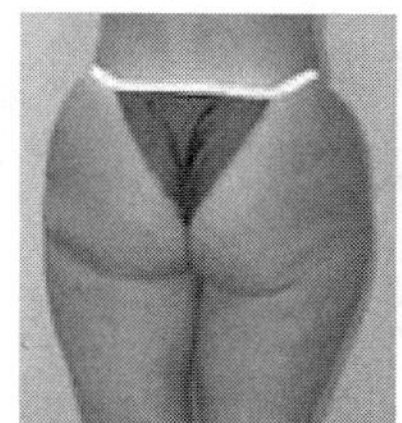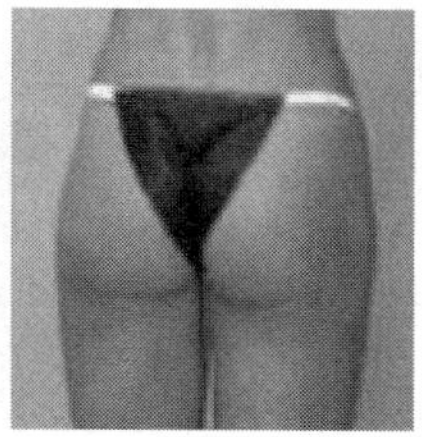

BEFORE   FIGURE 6-26   AFTER
LIPOSUCTION OF HIPS, THIGHS, & BUTTOCKS
ACTUAL PATIENT

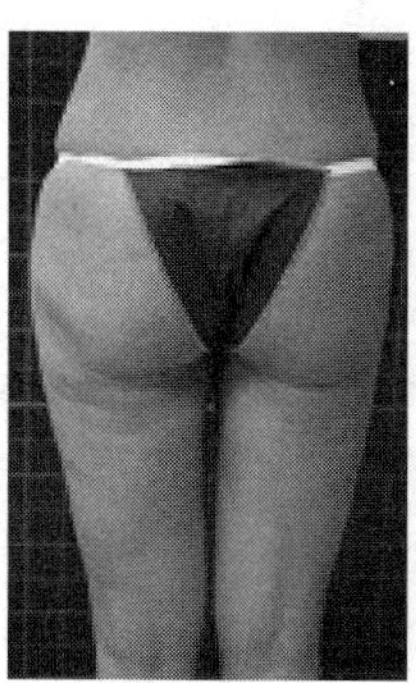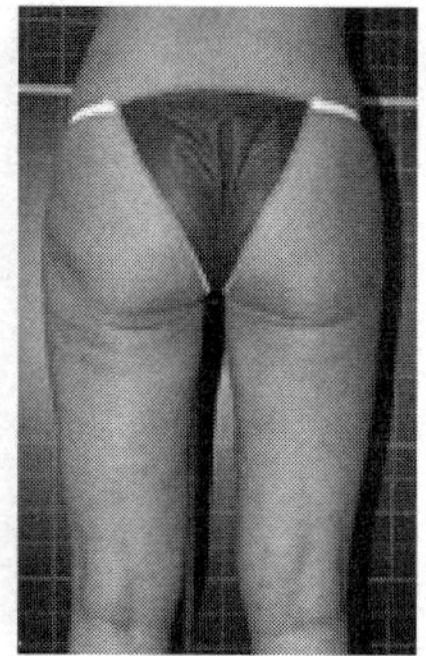

BEFORE   FIGURE 6-27   AFTER
LIPOSUCTION OF HIPS AND THIGHS
ACTUAL PATIENT

The outer thigh should be treated in conjunction with the area just below the buttocks (*inferior lateral*) and the upper posterior thighs.

Not addressing the fat in these other areas can make them disproportionate, and not aesthetically pleasing.

A patient might only request liposuction of the thighs but, to achieve optimal cosmetic results, the hips may need treatment as well.

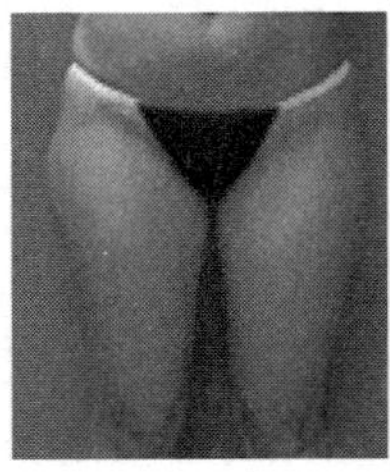 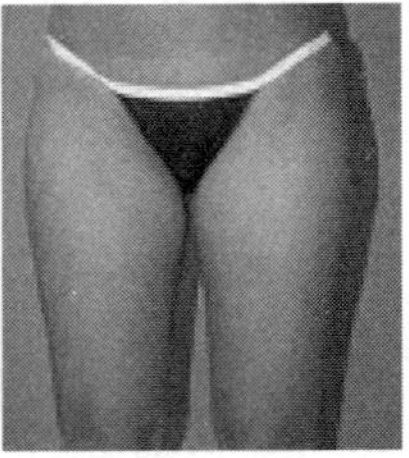

BEFORE   FIGURE 6-28   AFTER
LIPOSUCTION OF INNER AND OUTER THIGHS
ACTUAL PATIENT

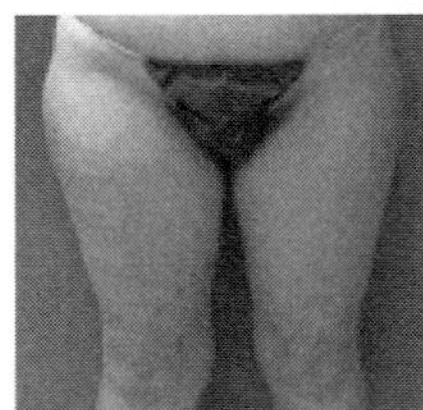 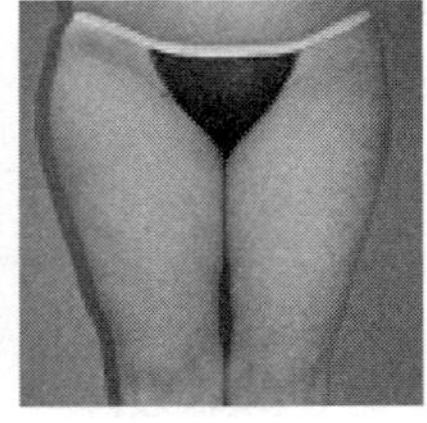

BEFORE   FIGURE 6-29   AFTER
LIPOSUCTION OF INNER AND OUTER THIGHS
ACTUAL PATIENT

Some surgeons attempt liposuction around the entire circumference of the thighs in a single treatment, which can cause inflammation and swelling, resulting in a lengthy recovery. Inflammation can impair absorption of the fluids infused during tumescent liposuction, leading to swelling of the legs and feet. That swelling can affect drainage from the legs, increasing the risk of deep vein thrombosis.

I aggressively address the inner and outer thighs, which respond well to fat withdrawal. I'm extremely conservative working in the front and back thigh, areas less able to tolerate liposuction.

Liposuction of the inner thigh can significantly improve the silhouette of the leg and eliminate rubbing of the thighs while walking.

To achieve symmetry, liposuction of the inner thighs should be done along with the inner knees, since most fat extends down to the knee area. With attention to these details, an experienced physician can consistently achieve outstanding results.

Patients with good skin elasticity get the best inner-thigh liposuction results. Older women and those who have lost an extensive amount of weight will see more limited improvement.

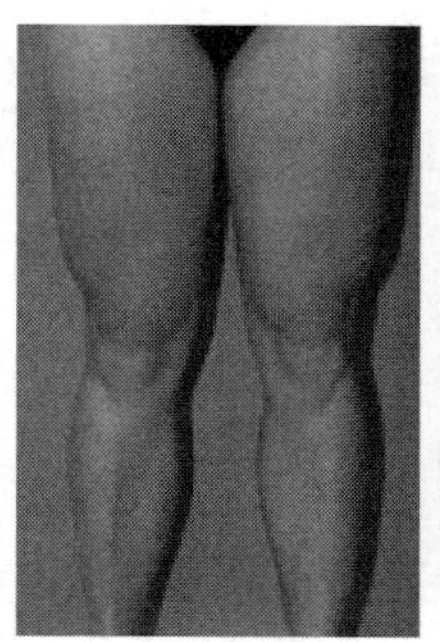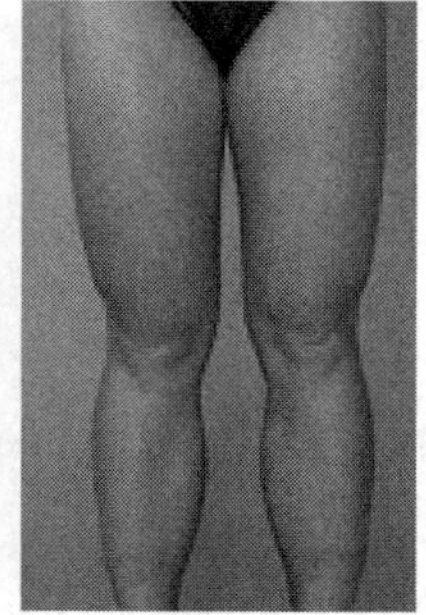

BEFORE   FIGURE 6-30   AFTER
LIPOSUCTION OF INNER & OUTER THIGHS,
(EXTREMELY FIT)
ACTUAL PATIENT

Facial Liposuction

Facial liposuction removes fatty deposits from those areas of the face — the chin, neck, and jowls — that can make a patient look older.

Facial liposuction using microcannulas offers a safe and effective treatment with virtually undetectable scars, plus rapid recovery. Frequently, facial liposuction can produce better results than other surgical techniques, since it gives a more natural appearance.

Liposuction can also be more cost-effective than a face lift. Cost varies from $2,000 to $5,000, and recovery time is between two and three days.

Patients with localized fat deposits in the face or neck are good candidates for facial liposuction.

Older patients with more wrinkled skin often combine liposuction and resurfacing with a laser or chemical peel for optimal results.

Both men and women have facial liposuction because of the minimal recovery time and the natural results they can get.

Which Facial Areas Respond Best to Liposuction?

The answers are: cheeks, below the chin, the jowls and, in many cases, the neck.

- Cheeks
  Some patients inherit a tendency to store excess fat here, giving the appearance of "chipmunk cheeks." The cheeks respond well to liposuction.
- Below the Chin
  The area just below the chin is prone to accumulation of fat, and a common complaint of patients. This area can be treated successfully, with favorable results.
- Jowls
  Fat can accumulate in the jowls: the lower cheeks along the jaw line. Fat causes a loss of definition, aging the face. Removing the fat deposits can take years off one's appearance.
- Neck
  Liposuction can improve a neck that has underlying fat, provided the patient has good skin elasticity. The procedure can create a well-defined angle to the chin and neck.

Recovery from facial liposuction is relatively quick. Patients can expect mild discomfort with some bruising and swelling. This should subside in two to three days.

Most facial liposuction patients return to normal activities within a week, and see the full results in three to six months. Cost for this procedure varies from $2,000 to $5,000.

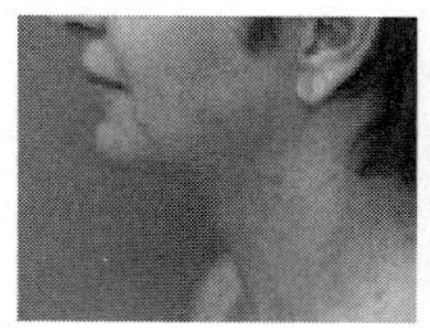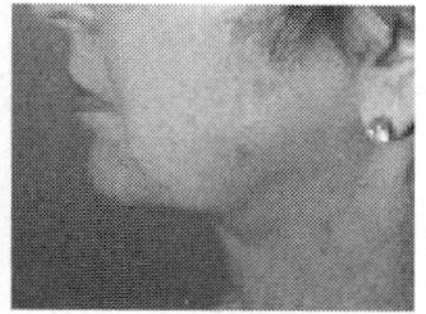

BEFORE   FIGURE 6-31   AFTER
LIPOSCULPTURE OF NECK & JOWLS
ACTUAL PATIENT IN HER 50s

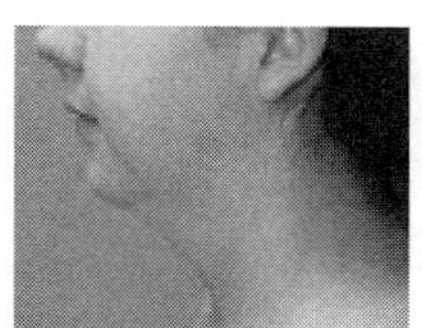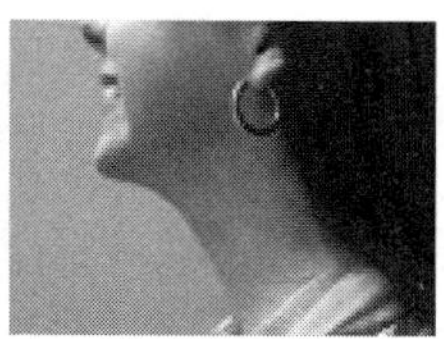

BEFORE   FIGURE 6-32   AFTER
LIPOSCULPTURE OF NECK AND JOWLS
ACTUAL PATIENT

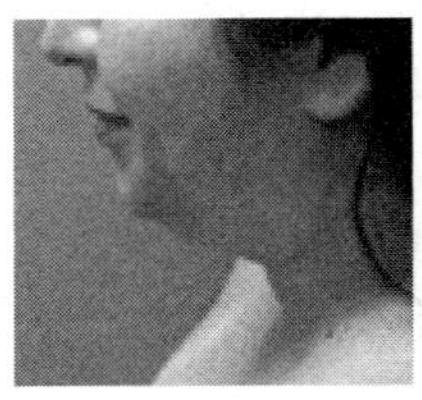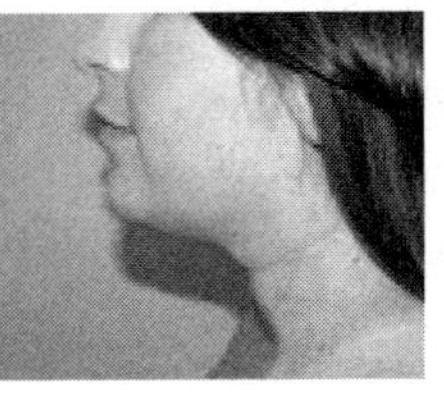

BEFORE   FIGURE 6-33   AFTER
ACTUAL PATIENT

7

"Real" Men Can Have Liposuction, Too

FAT COLLECTS IN different places on men's and women's bodies, which most of us know all too well. I won't go into detail about the research, but the differences in male and female fat distribution have been studied extensively.

Fat accumulation varies by age and race, as well as by gender. The older we get, the more the subcutaneous (just under the skin) fat decreases, and intra-abdominal fat increases. In other words, fat is found deeper within body tissue.

After about age thirty, the way fat accumulates (and where) is a product of genetics. Localized accumulations of this type of fat can be impossible to lose through exercise or dieting. Liposuction is effective on these resistant areas, and is a practical means of significantly changing the body's silhouette.

Fat Accumulation: The Differences between Male and Female Bodies

To better understand the differences in liposuction procedures for men and women, you first need to know the types of fat that male and female bodies store, and where it accumulates.

Women: The Pear Shape

Fat cells tend to congregate in the abdominal area of young women. This is the body's way of providing protection for a baby during pregnancy. Unfortunately, abdominal skin sags after giving birth, so fat deposits become more noticeable.

Women are also more likely than men to accumulate fat in the outer thighs, buttocks, hips, and torso, giving the female body what's called a *pear shape,* shown in Figure 7-1.

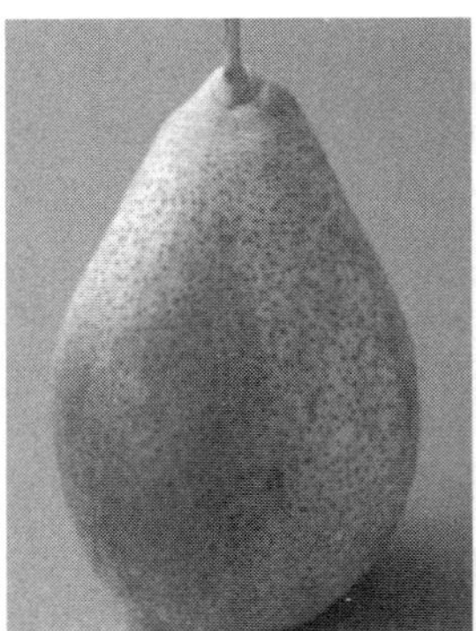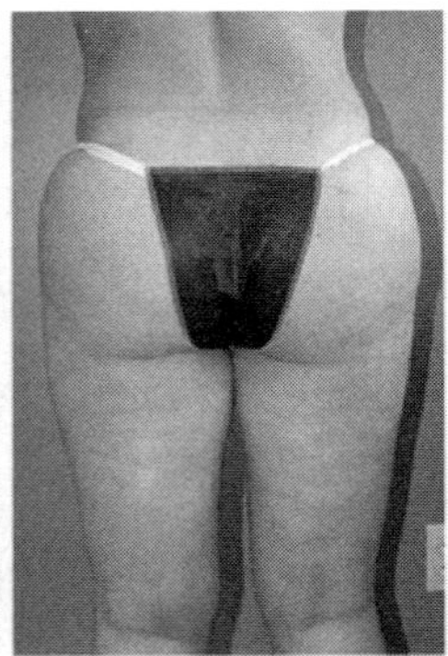

FIGURE 7-1
THE PEAR SHAPE

In women, fatty tissue in the abdominal and thigh area tends to be more superficial than deep, and is loose and easy to pinch. It breaks up well during liposuction.

It's important to note here that stretch marks in both men and women aren't correctable by liposuction. Stretch marks afflict the outer skin layer (the epidermis) which remains untouched in liposuction procedures. Consequently, there will be no change in their appearance.

Men: The Apple Shape — A Different Ballgame

Male patients who want to improve their overall appearance commonly request liposuction to sculpt specific areas of their bodies. But fat is more dense in men and harder to remove. This is especially true of fat in the chest area.

Men can develop fat around the torso and abdomen, as well as the chest area, giving their bodies what's known as the *apple shape,* shown in Figure 7-2.

You may be more familiar with its identifiable characteristics: "beer belly" and "love handles". Liposculpture can help maintain and even enhance a masculine appearance.

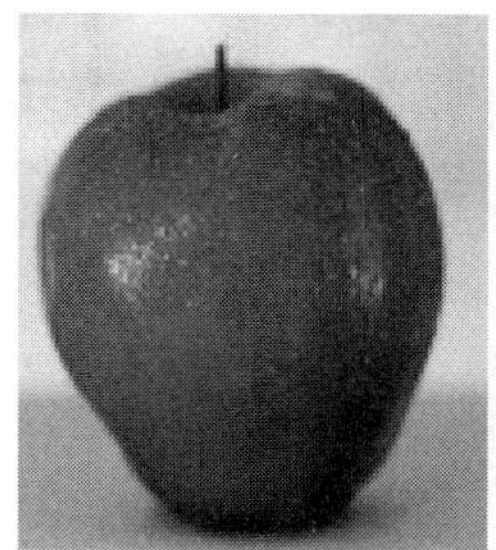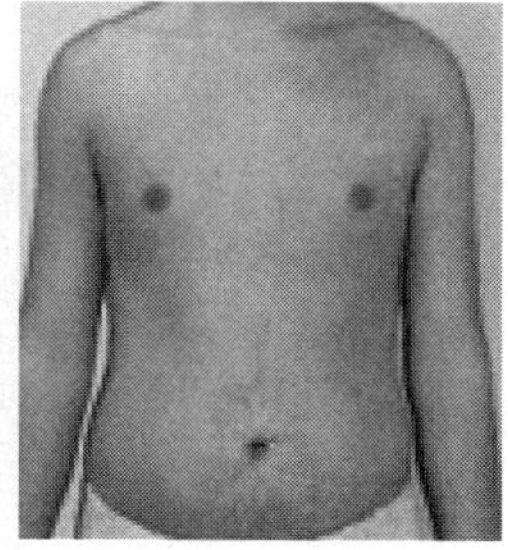

FIGURE 7-2
THE APPLE SHAPE

Some fat in men is stored intra-abdominally (under the muscle), so it can't be eliminated with liposuction. In that situation, significant improvement can only be made with a consistent diet and exercise plan.

The Benefits of Liposuction on the Male Body

According to the American Society for Aesthetic Plastic Surgery (ASAPS) in 2009, fifteen percent of all liposuction procedures performed in the United States were performed on men.

In my practice, a full 50 percent of the patients I see for liposuction are men. The main reason is this: There is significantly less "down-time" after liposuction than with more invasive procedures, so more men are choosing to refine and refresh their appearance through liposculpture.

The Cost of Male Liposuction Procedures

Some surgeons charge slightly more for liposuction procedures performed on men. There are three reasons:

First, fat on the male physique is generally more fibrous than in women, so it's more difficult and time-consuming to remove.

Second, men usually request liposuction of areas naturally more fibrous, such as the chest, love handles, and abdomen.

Third, men are typically larger than women, so liposuction often involves the treatment of a larger area than in a female.

The cost of liposuction to these areas ranges from $2,000 to $4,000 and recovery time is from three to five days.

Why Opt for Liposuction?

In spite of following a regimen of good diet and exercise, many men have difficulty losing fat in the flank area (*love handles*).

Liposuction can be extremely effective in reducing the appearance of love handles as well as the abdomen, another area notoriously difficult to tone.

The flanks lie on each side of the torso, between the middle of the ribcage and the hip. Liposuction can greatly improve the appearance of the flanks, and helps reduce abdominal bulge.

Eliminating Love Handles

Liposuction of the flanks is performed under local anesthetic so that the patient can roll over to allow the surgeon access to the back of the flanks.

Surgery is performed both vertically and horizontally. Continuing liposuction into the hip area helps create a more masculine profile, shown in Figure 7-3.

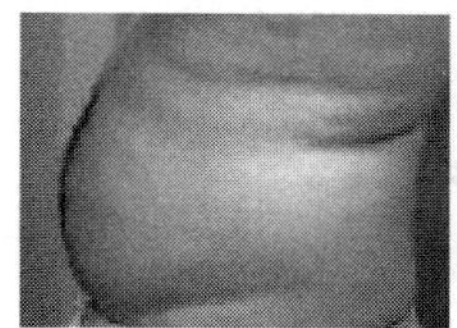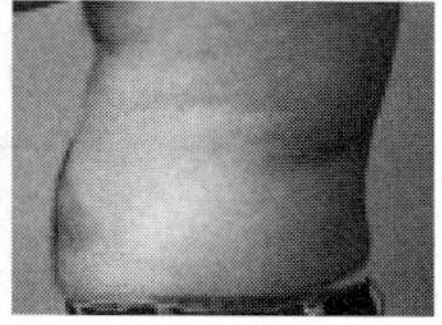

BEFORE   FIGURE 7-3   AFTER
MICROLIPO OF UPPER & LOWER ABDOMEN, LOVE HANDLES, &
FLANKS
ACTUAL 50-YEAR-OLD PATIENT

The surgeon must maintain a smooth and even transition from one area to the next, contouring carefully. After liposuction of the love handles and flanks, a patient may require additional procedures in order to get the results he desires.

That wasn't the case in my patient in Figure 7-4. He had a muscular physique that simply needed some "tweaking", and was elated with his new body.

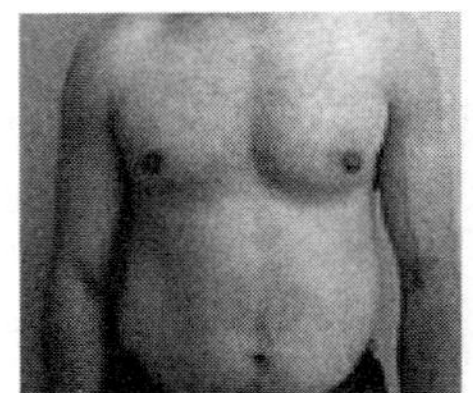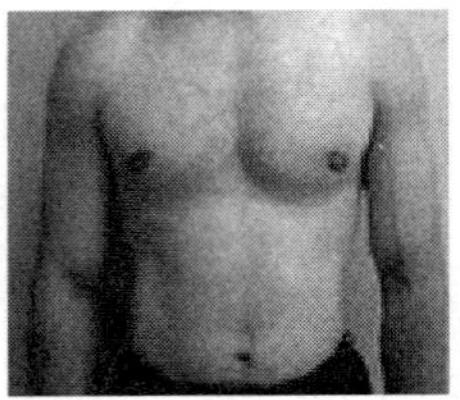

BEFORE   FIGURE 7-4   AFTER
MICROLIPO OF THE UPPER & LOWER ABDOMEN,
WAIST, & FLANKS
ACTUAL 30-YEAR-OLD PATIENT

Liposuction of Male Breasts

Liposuction can also be used for male breast reduction, but the surgeon must first determine whether the excess breast tissue is fatty or glandular. If the breast is primarily fatty tissue, liposuction is excellent for reducing breast size and improving the appearance of the chest.

Immediately following this procedure, my patient in Figure 7-5 already had more definition in the chest area.

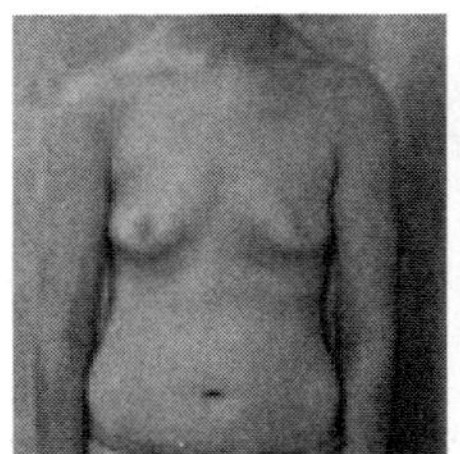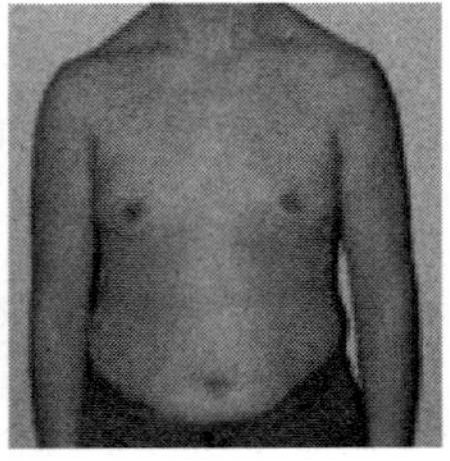

BEFORE   FIGURE 7-5   AFTER
ACTUAL PATIENT

Breast reduction surgery is more common for men than you might think. Over 40 percent of men are afflicted with gynecomastia (translated, "female breasts"), a condition in which firm breast tissue forms (See Figure 7-6).

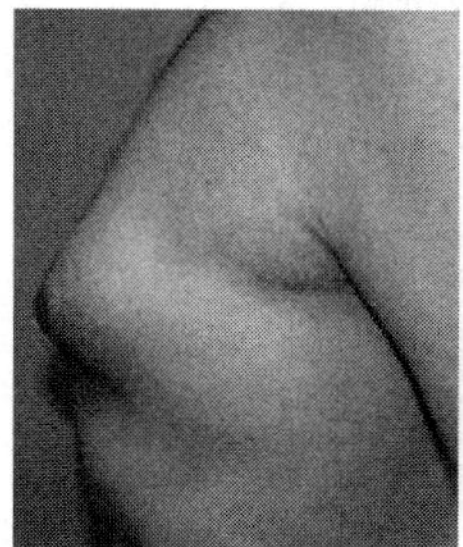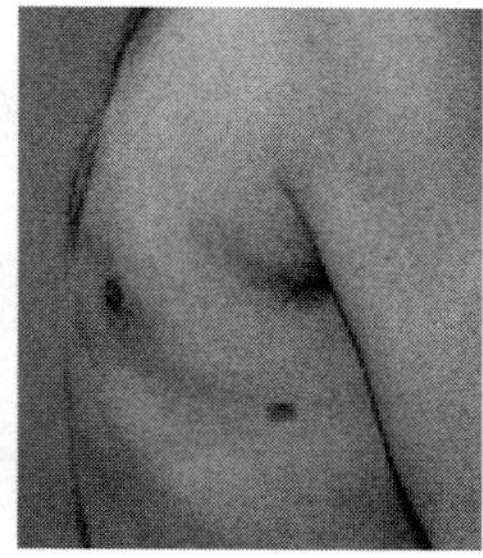

BEFORE   FIGURE 7-6   AFTER
ACTUAL PATIENT

Gynecomastia is usually caused by changes in hormone levels, and can occur as part of the aging process, when testes activity decreases.

Gynecomastia is seen most often when a male enters puberty. During the body's transition to manhood, there may be a temporary lag in the production of testosterone, so estrogen (present in every man) can cause breasts to develop.

It's estimated that approximately 65 percent of 14-year-old boys develop this condition; it disappears in 90 percent of them within 18 months to three years, without any treatment. I've been able to help many patients whose conditions don't improve naturally.

A man's dissatisfaction with the appearance of his breasts is subjective. Where one man sees no female characteristics in his physique, another may be quite self-conscious with even a minimal amount of gynecomastia.

The patient shown in Figure 7-7 was concerned with the appearance of his chest, and ecstatic with the results.

Male Breast Reduction was performed using liposuction. He says the procedure changed his life. To some observers, he had no problem to begin with, but it was important to his self-esteem to have the procedure.

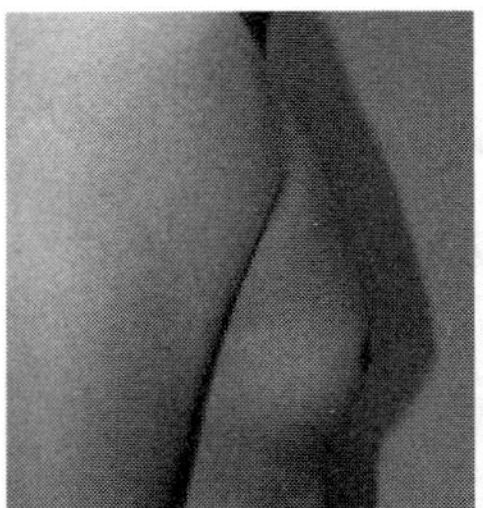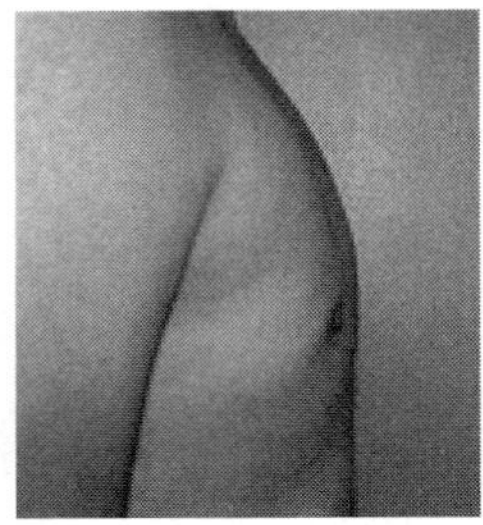

BEFORE   FIGURE 7-7   AFTER
ACTUAL PATIENT

Men undergoing treatment for prostate or testicular cancer are often given estrogen as part of their treatment, resulting in gynecomastia. Other causes include alcoholism, HIV infection, renal failure treated with dialysis, and reactions to certain drug therapies.

Understandably, gynecomastia can cause embarrassment. Reluctant to discuss it, men are likely to hide their condition.

They avoid participating in any activity where their chests would be exposed. Once the unwanted breast tissue is removed, confidence is increased significantly.

Consider my patient in Figure 7-8. His breasts were feminine in shape; with the reduction in tissue, his profile is vastly improved.

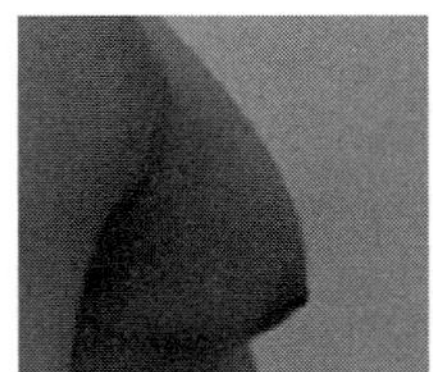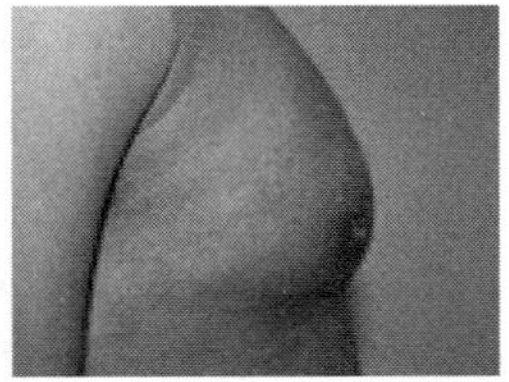

BEFORE   FIGURE 7-8   AFTER
ACTUAL PATIENT

If the breasts are asymmetrical or oddly shaped, the patient should be examined for possible tumors prior to any surgical intervention, after which the surgeon can determine the best course of action.

Pseudo-gynecomastia is the accumulation of fat (rather than breast tissue) in the breast area. This can occur with age and/or weight gain, and is easily resolved with liposuction.

I'm one of the few surgeons performing liposuction for male breast reduction (with over 1,000 to date), with excellent results. The cost for this procedure varies from $2,000 to $5,000 with recovery time between two and three days.

Figures 7-9 through 7-13 show the improvements my patients achieved when I performed liposuction on their chests.

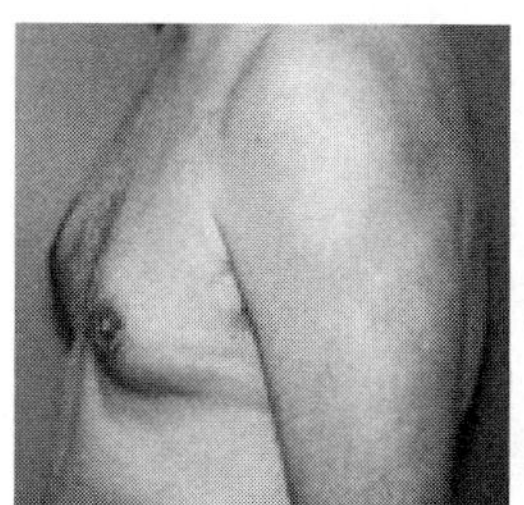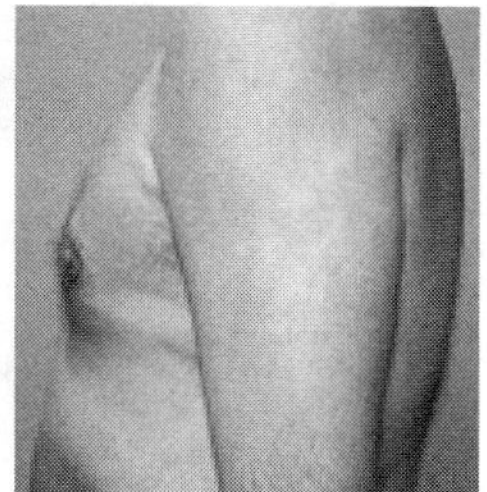

BEFORE   FIGURE 7-9   AFTER
BREAST REDUCTION USING MICROLIPO
ACTUAL PATIENT

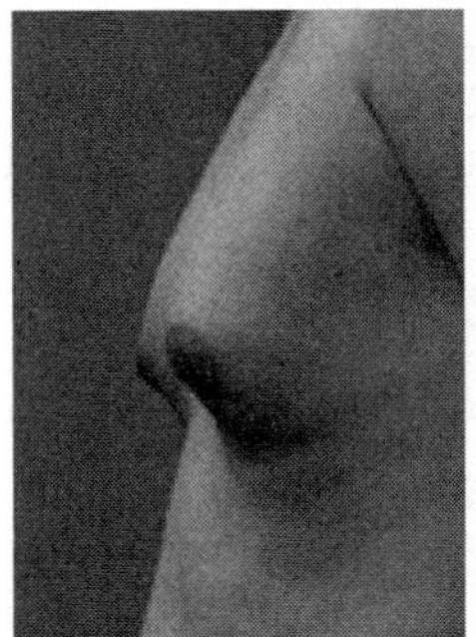 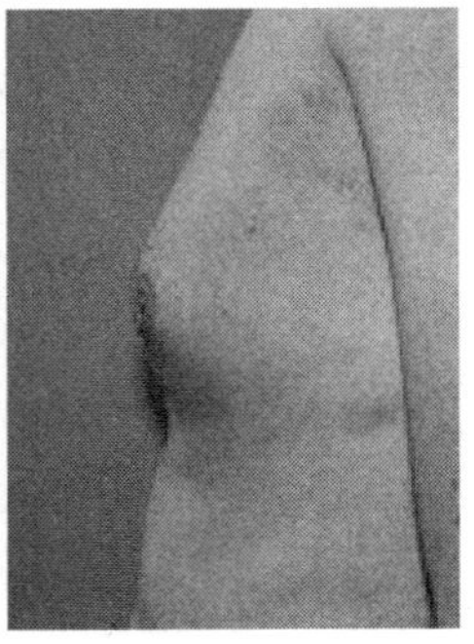

BEFORE   FIGURE 7-10   AFTER
ACTUAL PATIENT

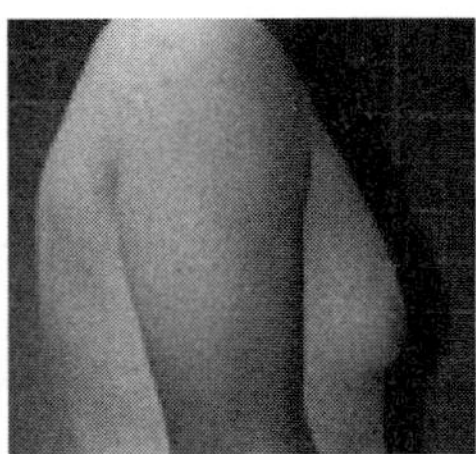 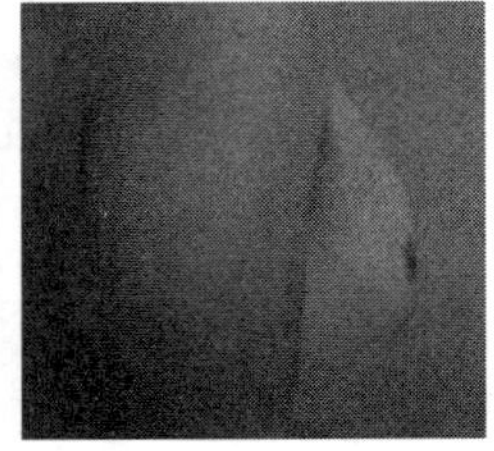

BEFORE   FIGURE 7-11   AFTER
ACTUAL PATIENT

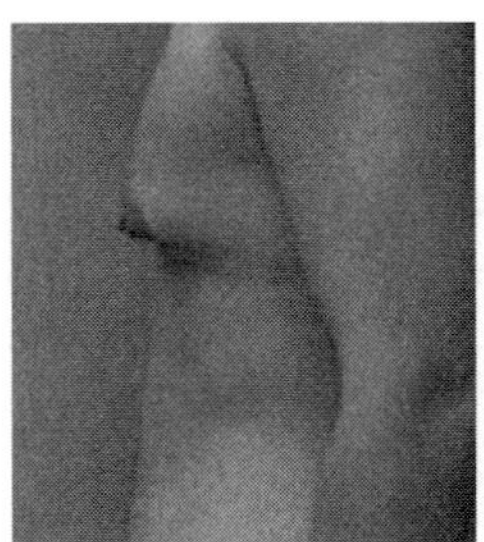 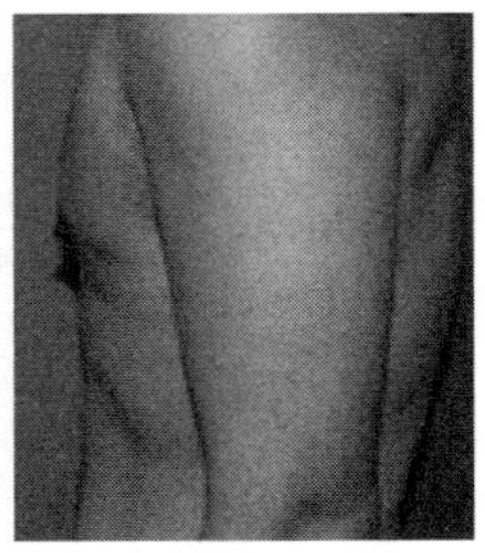

BEFORE   FIGURE 7-12   AFTER
ACTUAL PATIENT

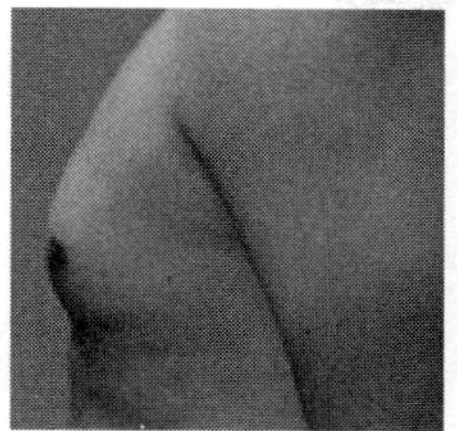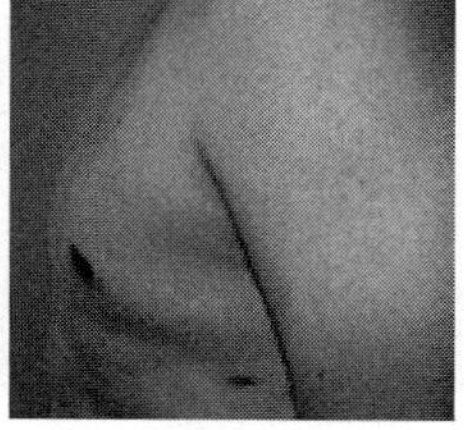

BEFORE   FIGURE 7-13   AFTER
ACTUAL PATIENT

Because I've helped hundreds of patients lead more fulfilled lives using techniques I've developed especially for male breast reduction, I'm frequently asked to speak at international medical conferences to share my innovative approach to this procedure.

8 | What to Anticipate: Surgery and Recovery

THOUGH LIPOSUCTION HAS become a common procedure, it's still surgery. Anxiety about your impending surgery can be alleviated if you do your research and take a proactive role in the recovery process.

The following information will guide you in preparing for surgery and explain what to expect afterwards.

Realistic Expectations

Once the decision has been made to proceed with liposuction, it's important that a patient has realistic expectations and understands the limitations of the procedure. In this chapter, I'll explain in detail what can be expected, and give answers to common questions my patients have asked.

Liposuction is the permanent removal of fat cells. It isn't a cure-all; a patient still needs to maintain a balanced diet and exercise regimen following the procedure. Minor weight gain shouldn't affect the areas treated.

However, a significant amount of weight gained will give the treated areas a fuller appearance, since there are still some fat cells remaining.

Remember, liposuction isn't meant for weight loss; it simply contours and sculpts the body. Many women also opt for liposuction to improve the appearance of cellulite.

While there's no guarantee that liposuction will produce perfection in the eyes of the patient, a skilled, experienced surgeon will provide the best results possible.

Cellulite

Most females are afflicted with "cottage cheese" on the thighs, midsection, and arms, otherwise known as cellulite. The majority of liposuction patients achieve an amazing 50 percent improvement in skin firmness and texture, if not more.

To understand how such phenomenal results can be achieved, you need to understand the nature of cellulite. Cellulite is an accumulation of fat, fluid, and toxins trapped into a hardened network of fibers in the deep levels of the skin. This area benefits tremendously from liposuction. While liposuction doesn't eliminate cellulite completely, it can help delay deterioration of the tissue, a major component in the aging process.

Stress, poor diet, lack of exercise, genetics, and hormones all have a hand in determining the degree of cellulite a person has. Treatment procedures vary from water therapy to laser massage to electric muscle stimulation to liposuction. In my opinion, liposuction is by far the most effective and long-term treatment.

As with any medical procedure, communication between doctor and patient is vital before undergoing liposuction. The physician you select should explain in detail both the surgery and the possible side effects.

Ask questions so that you're informed and comfortable with both your surgeon and the procedure. If you have further questions after the consultation, the physician's office staff should be able to give you answers. But don't hesitate to schedule another appointment with the doctor if you have any lingering concerns.

Preparation

You and your surgeon will have an in-depth consultation prior to the procedure. This should include detailed information about the procedure from start to finish, as well as its risks and limitations.

The physician and his staff will tell you specifically what to do prior to surgery. He'll discuss the anesthesia he intends to use, answer questions about the facility where the liposuction procedure will take place, go over the costs involved in the procedure, and give you a list of medications and supplies to purchase and have on hand before the procedure.

Some basic precautions he'll discuss include discontinuing all forms of aspirin, as well as any medication and vitamins that could interfere with the ability of the blood to clot effectively.

Excessive bleeding is a very real side effect of aspirin-containing medications, so it's important to follow your doctor's orders.

If you smoke, you'll be required to stop smoking entirely for at least two weeks before liposuction and at least two weeks after.

Smoking decreases the blood supply to vessels and capillaries, and interferes with the healing process.

The day before surgery, pack a bag with loose, comfortable clothing to return home in, and arrange transportation to and from the facility. Try to get adequate sleep the night before the procedure.

You must fast and refrain from drinking any liquids (even water) from midnight on, to avoid nausea before or during the procedure.

Surgery Day

On the day of the liposuction procedure, shower with an antibacterial soap (usually provided by your doctor), and arrive at the surgical facility wearing no makeup or nail polish.

Upon arrival, you'll sign a consent form stating that you understand the risks, benefits, possible outcomes, and all liposuction alternatives.

Your surgeon should have discussed this in detail during the consultation appointment. Signing the consent form also signifies that all your questions were answered before the procedure.

The physician will instruct you on post-operative care before he begins, to make sure you understand how to treat the surgical areas to help the healing process.

Once all forms are completed and explanations given, the surgeon will administer medication to eliminate anxiety and help control your blood pressure during the procedure.

The surgeon will take "before" pictures of the targeted areas to compare with the post-operative results. The areas to be treated will then be marked on your body.

In case you're wondering, the pictures taken are used to guide the surgeon in performing the procedure. While liposuction procedures are relatively standard, every person is different. The surgeon customizes the procedure to meet each patient's specific needs.

The Procedure

You'll be helped onto an operating table and kept warm, and your skin will be sterilized. In most cases, a member of the surgical staff connects the patient to monitoring devices which relay information such as blood pressure, oxygen saturation levels, and heart rate during surgery. An IV may be inserted to administer medications.

With few exceptions, general anesthesia isn't required for liposuction. That means no nausea, an unpleasant aspect of any procedure.

If minimal sedation is used, extensive monitoring isn't usually necessary. Once you're comfortably sedated, the incision sites are injected with local anesthetic by syringe.

Small (one to two millimeter) incisions are made to introduce tiny cannulas which bathe the treatment area with tumescent anesthetic fluid.

The size of a liposuction incision is 1-2 mm and is commonly left open to improve drainage, to speed recovery time by reducing swelling and bruising. It's also been reported that infection rates are much lower than when the incisions are closed with sutures.

Fat is dissolved with ultrasound, laser, or other devices to decrease the size of the fat cells and dislodge them from the surrounding tissue. A suction cannula moves the fat from deeper tissue to a more superficial level.

Symmetry of the area is determined from all angles by the surgeon and other operating room personnel. Once your surgeon is satisfied that the treatment area is improved to his satisfaction, the area will be cleaned with a sterile solution.

Compression Garments

Compression garments are essential to recovery after liposuction. They apply pressure to the treated area to keep the tissue from shifting as the patient moves.

They aid in the prevention of blood clots and pockets of blood (*seromas*) that can form. Compression garments also help control pain and swelling, and help the body adjust to its new shape.

A compression garment will be fitted to you immediately after surgery. A foam insert may be used under the garment to reduce the possibility of blood or other fluids collecting (and decrease bruising).

You'll be under observation after surgery until your vital signs are stable and you're ambulatory. You won't be discharged until these criteria are met.

It's recommended that you have someone stay with you overnight after surgery. This person can monitor you, make sure you drink fluids and eat as instructed, as well as help you to and from the bathroom.

There may be considerable drainage from the incision sites so to protect your pillow and bed, put a thick towel, old shower curtain, or even a painter's drop cloth between you and the sheets, or use a trash bag under the sheets to keep fluid from getting to your mattress. A plastic bag under the pillow case will keep drainage (from facial or chin incisions) from soiling the pillow.

Recovery

With today's liposuction techniques, recovery is much faster and less painful than ever before. Liposuction is usually an outpatient procedure, and patients can be sent home within hours after surgery is completed. In most cases, patients are able to return to normal activities within two to three days.

Post-Operative Care

Liposuction post-operative care focuses on minimizing risk while optimizing results. These are my recommendations for a faster recovery:

- Avoid alcohol
- Wear the compression garment for the length of time prescribed
- Stay hydrated
- Avoid exposing the liposuction area to drastic temperature changes, like when using ice packs or heating pads

- Keep post-operative appointments to help the surgeon monitor your healing
- Avoid strenuous activities for several weeks (as determined by your doctor), until the incisions heal
- No heavy lifting (over 20 pounds), aerobic exercise, swimming, contact sports, tennis, or golf for several weeks after the surgery (as determined by your doctor)
- Get up and walk as soon as possible after surgery, and continue to move frequently over the coming weeks to reduce swelling and prevent blood clots from forming
- Do *NOT* apply hydrogen peroxide or plastic bandages to the incision sites; they need to drain freely
- Stand up slowly from any sitting position after surgery to reduce the risk of fainting
- Remove compression garments slowly. Sit down immediately if you get dizzy or lightheaded. Ideally, have help when you take your first shower after surgery

The First Two Weeks after Surgery

The vast majority of patients are able to move and walk within a day or two after liposuction. The compression garment will be worn for several days after the procedure, to help in recovery.

Few patients report notable pain the day after liposuction. Usually the discomfort is minor and can be relieved with medication, or walking to reduce soreness.

In the first days after tumescent liposuction, the anesthetic solution from surgery drains from the incisions. This drainage helps healing and reduces recovery time. Bandages will be changed within the first forty-eight hours.

Transition to a secondary garment that is less restrictive, as directed by your surgeon. These are available at most department stores or online retailers, as mentioned in Chapter 1.

Patients are usually prescribed 3-14 days of pain medication, but most don't need it. If you experience severe pain following liposuction, notify your physician immediately.

You should shower rather than bathe for one week after liposuction. Incisions remain open for that amount of time, so taking showers reduces the risk of infection.

Recovery from liposuction can be a bit uncomfortable, but most patients are back to work within a few days.

Patients can experience discomfort, burning, swelling, and temporary numbness in the treated area. Medications can alleviate the discomfort, and wearing a body compression garment helps minimize swelling.

Don't be surprised if you experience post-operative "blues". You may wonder: why in the world did I do this to myself?

There are several reasons for what you're feeling: anesthesia wearing off so you have more pain than anticipated, disappointment with your immediate post-op appearance (remember, it takes some time for swelling and bruising to resolve), and impatience with the healing process. These are all normal feelings.

I recommend keeping a journal beginning the day of your procedure. Every day, look for improvements, no matter how slight, and enter them into your diary.

When you start to feel like you're not progressing, go back and read a few pages. It's amazing how much improvement you'll remember.

Exercise

It's extremely important to refrain from excessive exercise for at least one week after surgery. You can usually begin walking within two days of the procedure, and slowly work back into a normal exercise routine. The key to optimal recovery is to take things slowly and follow your doctor's instructions.

When to Expect the Final Results

The treated area should tighten to the degree of the patient's skin elasticity. Swelling gradually diminishes following liposuction, with final results noticeable by the sixth month. The important thing to remember is not to expect to see the final results immediately.

If a large area has been treated or a significant amount of fat has been removed, liposuction recovery time will be longer.

Swelling and bruising will gradually disappear within one to three months. During that time, it may be difficult to see any improvements. Skin in the treated area needs to adjust to fit the new, more slender tissue beneath the surface.

It's important to remember that results aren't just aesthetic; liposuction is often the first step toward a healthier, more active lifestyle for patients.

Your surgeon will encourage you to exercise regularly and follow a well-balanced diet, in order to maintain your new body shape. You'll gradually find yourself less self-conscious at the gym or health club. Maybe you'll take a healthy diet more seriously, or adopt a more aggressive exercise regime.

Don't assume that because liposuction permanently removes fat cells, it's impossible to regain weight in the treated areas. That's only partially true.

Remember, we're born with a fixed number of fat cells, and liposuction removes only some of those cells. Those remaining can still swell as they absorb fat from food, especially if you don't exercise or follow a healthy diet. Substantial weight gain (or loss) after liposuction can cause rippling and skin irregularity.

A good understanding of what liposuction will and won't do is an important factor in determining whether or not the patient is a good candidate for surgery. I hope this has been helpful in bringing you one step closer to your decision about liposuction.

9

Possible Side Effects and Complications

ALTHOUGH LIPOSUCTION HAS proven to be as safe as it is effective, there are potential side effects, just as with any surgical procedure. Here are some situations patients commonly encounter after liposuction.

Common Conditions After Liposuction
Swelling
Swelling is caused by an accumulation of excess fluid in the treated tissue. This usually resolves within three weeks.

Bumps or Lumps
Bumps and lumps are seen when the treated area temporarily loses its shape or texture. Lumps can be caused by scar tissue forming unevenly. Massaging the area helps smooth these imperfections.

Bleeding
Bleeding (along with drainage of the infused fluid used during liposuction) from the incision site is normal.

Excessive bleeding can occur if aspirin, anti-inflammatory medication (like Anaprox® or Motrin®), and vitamin E aren't eliminated two weeks before surgery.

Hypersensitivity

Increased sensitivity around the liposuction treatment area is normal, typically subsiding in a few weeks. If pain continues or is excessive, contact your surgeon immediately.

Numbness

Liposuction can cause some numbness, rarely permanent. Numbness is not a sign of nerve damage. Massaging the area will help eliminate the numbness.

Scarring

Scarring occurs when fibrous tissue replaces normal surface tissue during healing. Surgical scars are permanent. However, tumescent liposuction is performed using a very small incision (less than ¼-inch in length) for each treatment area.

Incisions are made in natural skin creases, hidden in pubic hair, or made inside the belly button, so are virtually invisible, except on very close observation.

KELOID SCARRING

A keloid is thick, puckered scar tissue that grows beyond the edge of a wound or incision. Keloids are usually genetic, and affect some individuals and body areas more than others.

If the patient has a history of keloid scarring at previous incision sites, it's possible they'll develop at liposuction sites, as well. These scars aren't dangerous; they're just not especially attractive.

Stiffness

Stiffness is common when the patient doesn't move around enough after the liposuction procedure. The best solution is for the patient to be up and around, walking as soon as possible.

Bruising

We all know what a bruise is, but what causes it? Bruising is the result of blood pooling into subcutaneous tissue under the skin or in mucous membranes.

When there's no break in the skin for it to be released, blood becomes trapped inside, resulting in discoloration that goes through a variety of colors, from purple to black to green and finally to yellow, as the blood is absorbed through the natural healing process.

Contour Irregularities

Contour irregularities include dimpling, rippling, bagginess, and lumps. Most of these issues are improved with massage (the use of numbing creams, like those used for arthritis pain, are especially effective in reducing temporary discomfort during massage), external ultrasound, and exercise to help increase blood circulation.

Asymmetry

Asymmetry means that a patient's body is disproportionate: the left and right side of the body are different sizes or shapes. A skilled surgeon can produce uniform results even when a body is asymmetrical, and will be able to balance sides of a patient's body that become asymmetrical after liposuction. This usually involves a short "touch-up" visit.

Sagging Skin

Loose or thin skin, stretch marks, extensive sun exposure, and age contribute to the skin's failure to tighten after liposuction. The best liposuction results are achieved in healthy individuals of normal weight with firm, elastic skin.

Thrombophlebitis

Thrombophlebitis is a very rare condition that occurs when the blood clots in one or more veins, causing inflammation. Superficial thrombophlebitis affects veins near the skin surface, and deep thrombophlebitis affects deeper, larger veins. The areas affected are extremely small.

Thrombophlebitis usually responds well when diagnosed promptly.

Medications can help alleviate thrombophlebitis (analgesics, pain medications, or anti-inflammatory medications such as Ibuprofen), or support stockings and wraps can be worn to reduce discomfort.

The patient may be advised to:

- Elevate the affected area to reduce swelling
- Keep pressure off the area to reduce pain and decrease the risk of further damage
- Apply moist heat to reduce inflammation and pain

Swollen Ankles

Ankles can swell no matter what area of the body was treated with liposuction. Because of gravity, fluid flows south, so ankles receive the excess fluid buildup, manifested by swelling.

Rare Complications after Liposuction

According to studies, liposuction performed by board-certified cosmetic surgeons resulted in only a .03 percent complication rate.

In all my years of practice since 1973, I have encountered only 2 significant complications. Both involved pre-existing conditions that were not divulged by the patients.

According to a study by the American Society of Plastic Surgeons (ASPS), liposuction performed by board-certified plastic surgeons resulted in only a .03 percent complication rate.

Factors that can increase the risk of complications include:

- The use of general anesthesia for liposuction surgery
- Extracting more than six liters of tissue in one procedure, requiring increased anesthesia, administered over a longer period of time
- Extended length of surgery
- Multiple procedures performed in one surgery
- A patient with compromised pre-operative health

While liposuction is very safe when performed by skilled surgeons, it's important to know all the risks, including those which are extremely rare.

Any and all surgical procedures carry with them a possibility of death. Deaths related to liposuction surgery can occur for a number of reasons, some of which are:

- Formation of fatal blood clots
- Perforation of the abdominal wall or bowels
- Shock
- Hemodilution, caused by excessive fluid infused into the bloodstream during the procedure

Blood Clots

Blood clots (*deep venuous thrombosis*, or *DVT*) can form in the deep veins of the pelvis or legs after any surgery, including liposuction. Blood clots form after prolonged immobility (which underscores the importance of standing and moving regularly — at least once an hour — after surgery).

To increase circulation after liposuction surgery, make a conscious effort to keep blood flowing in the legs by flexing the feet frequently, even while seated or laying down. Blood clots can form if the blood pools for too long in any one area.

Perforation of Vital Organs

Perforation of vital organs (for example, abdominal wall or bowels) can occur during liposuction. The surgeon has a limited visual field during surgery, so a large portion of the procedure is done through palpation: feeling gently with the fingertips. This requires focused attention and skill.

Choosing a surgeon experienced in liposuction greatly reduces the risk of this complication.

Shock

Shock is the body's natural reaction to trauma. It becomes a medical emergency when the organs and tissues of the body don't receive adequate blood flow, depriving them of oxygen (carried in the blood). This can result in serious damage or even death.

To prevent shock, the surgeon should introduce only enough fluid necessary for the liposuction procedure, and never remove more than the recommended amount of fat (I remove no more than 4 liters) at one time.

Liposuction of more than 6 liters of fat is considered Mega-Lipo, and must take place in a hospital.

Hemodilution

Hemodilution is caused by an increase in the fluid content of blood, resulting in a lowered concentration of necessary nutrients.

Hemodilution can occur if a patient has excessive amounts of fluid injected and extreme amounts of fat and body fluid removed (over 6 liters).

Lidocaine Toxicity

The use of lidocaine poses particular hazards, especially since experts haven't yet determined safe injectable levels. Individuals with limited liver function or those who drink alcohol to excess may not be able to metabolize lidocaine effectively. Consequently, lidocaine toxicity is a concern.

Most surgeons err on the side of caution, and introduce minimal amounts rather than put the patient at risk by using too much lidocaine.

Infection

Open drainage of the liposuction incisions lessens the risk of infection, but infection can occur following any surgical procedure.

It's important for the patient to follow the post-operative instructions for wound care. If excessive redness or pain develops, the patient should contact the surgeon immediately.

Seromas

Seromas aren't the same as hematomas (which contain red blood cells) or abscesses (which are caused by infection and contain pus).

When small blood vessels are ruptured, fluid can seep out. This clear fluid collects in a pocket (called a seroma) under the skin after surgery.

The excess fluid contained in a seroma needs to be drained by the surgeon. There can also be inflammation, caused by dying injured cells.

The fluid gradually absorbs (often taking many days or weeks) but can leave a knot under the skin.

Allergic Reactions

Certain drug interactions can be life-threatening so any adverse reaction to medication or anesthesia used during a liposuction procedure can be very serious.

It's important that the patient tell the surgeon about allergies or reactions to medications, as well as any medication presently being taken (including over-the-counter and herbal supplements).

Problems Caused by Excessive Liposuction

There are risks associated with removing too much fat from targeted areas at once, as well as having excessive liposuction performed in a single surgical session.

In order to minimize surgical complications and the side effects of overexposure to anesthesia, patients should schedule large liposuction procedures several days apart.

Some of the more minor liposuction problems a patient can experience include dents, lumps, and loose skin. Dents can be corrected by fat transfer if necessary, while lumps can be massaged away, and excess skin excised.

Secondary Lipo –
Revisions of Other Surgeons' Work

Patients who have had previous liposuction procedures performed by other surgeons are sometimes unhappy with the results.

No one should settle for a poor result. Revision surgeries take experience and skill. I'm what you'd call a "factory-trained and tested" surgeon, performing very difficult revisions at least twice a week, and have provided excellent outcomes for my patients.

The moral of the story: select a qualified surgeon who performs these procedures often.

Avoiding Possible Side Effects of Liposuction

Certain medical conditions (such as diabetes) can affect healing and cause adverse effects. The best way to minimize the possibility of side effects is for the patient to provide as complete a medical history as possible to the surgeon, as well as a list of prescription and over-the-counter drugs, vitamins, or natural herbs being taken.

In preparation for liposuction, the patient will have a physical examination to evaluate overall health. That assures the doctor that the procedure can be performed safely.

Smoking affects the body's ability to heal by causing constriction of blood vessels. The patient must stop smoking at least two weeks prior to surgery and two weeks after, at a minimum.

Many surgeons refuse to perform surgery if a patient ignores this requirement.

Follow your doctor's instructions in regard to replacing the fluid lost during the procedure. I recommend that my patients drink Gatorade® or a similar product for at least 48 hours post-operatively, to replace electrolytes and restore the balance of fluids in the body.

The Weeks Following Liposuction

After liposuction, you'll be allowed to resume light exercise depending on the speed of your recovery. Exercise helps increase blood flow to all parts of the body, making the body heal faster.

Not only does exercise boost circulation, it also stimulates the skin to tighten. Start to slowly and gradually increase the intensity of your workouts.

Don't engage in strenuous exercise too soon after surgery; Sweating inside your compression garment could increase the risk of infection at the incision sites.

Minor liposuction complications, problems, and disappointment in general can be minimized by fully understanding the risks and benefits associated with liposuction, and having realistic expectations prior to undergoing the procedure.

A patient must do his part too, by following the doctor's orders before and after surgery.

It's extremely important to choose a cosmetic surgeon who explains the potential side effects and risks of liposuction. The surgeon should also be in good standing within the county's medical society, have extensive training in liposuction, and use state-of-the-art facilities.

Do your research, and interview several surgeons. Make your choice based on the criteria I've given, and you'll be adequately prepared for your liposuction procedure.

10

What Does the Future Hold?

THE MOST OBVIOUS signs of age are written on the face, when fat diminishes and skin loses its elasticity. While this breakdown is part of the natural aging process, it can also result from excessive squinting, frowning, and smiling.

Previously, the only way to erase time was with full-scale facial surgery, sometimes giving less-than-optimal results: tighter skin that didn't always look natural.

Enriched Cell-Assisted Lipotransfer (ECAL)

Enriched Cell-Assisted Lipotransfer or *ECAL* (stem-cell transfer) uses the body's own fat and the natural stem cells it contains to refresh and reinvigorate appearance.

Micro-grafting of stem-cell-rich fat has proven to be superior to injecting artificial fillers (such as Restylane®) for the re-creation of a youthful look.

Adult stem cells, found largely in adipose (fat) tissue, can help the body repair itself when transferred to target areas. This state-of-the-art technique in harvesting and fat-grafting provides optimal cosmetic results that last for years.

ECAL is a boon to modern plastic surgery. Cells are harvested from one area of the body and reintroduced to another, so aren't rejected. In a nutshell, chemicals or lasers aren't nearly as effective as ECAL.

Small amounts of fatty tissue and stem cells are micro-grafted into specific locations beneath the skin to rebuild new tissue structure. Stem cells, activated by the growth factors they contain, cause new blood vessels to grow, supporting the newly-grafted cells.

It's now possible to store current patients' own (autologous) fat and stem cells for future use when needed. This procedure can be performed on an outpatient basis with minimal anesthesia.

Fat containing high concentrations of stem cells can be withdrawn, processed, and injected into facial-contour soft tissue (e.g. cheekbones, nasal and mouth lines, around the eyes, etc.), where the stem cells tone, improve skin pigmentation and quality, and tighten pores.

Benefits of ECAL

- Downtime is reduced; healing takes place in a matter of days, rather than weeks
- Cost is roughly half that of a traditional face lift
- Skin texture is markedly improved, not achievable with a traditional face lift
- The surgeon can control the volume of cells introduced to the target area, giving more predictable results

Weekend Recovery Rejuva-lift ECAL results are more natural and superior to those achieved using artificial fillers. It can also be used to correct facial deformities as well as post-traumatic defects. Harvesting fat cells for transfer is often performed in conjunction with other procedures, such as liposuction.

Before and after photos of one of my patients, a 40-year-old horsewoman, are shown in Figure 10-1. Her skin had sustained substantial wind and sun damage. ECAL enhances both skin quality and the underlying contours of the face. You can see the exciting and remarkable improvement in her skin texture and tightness.

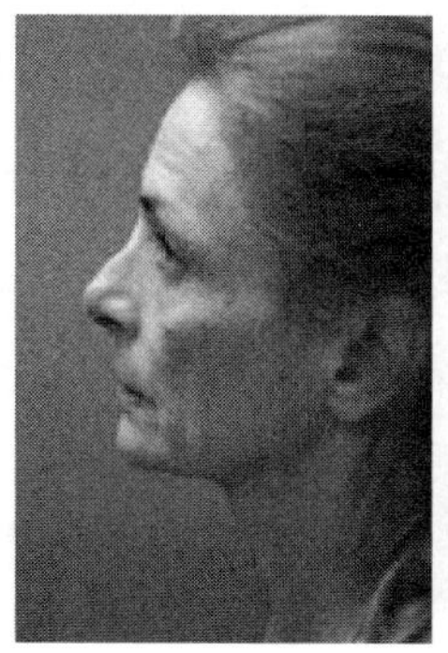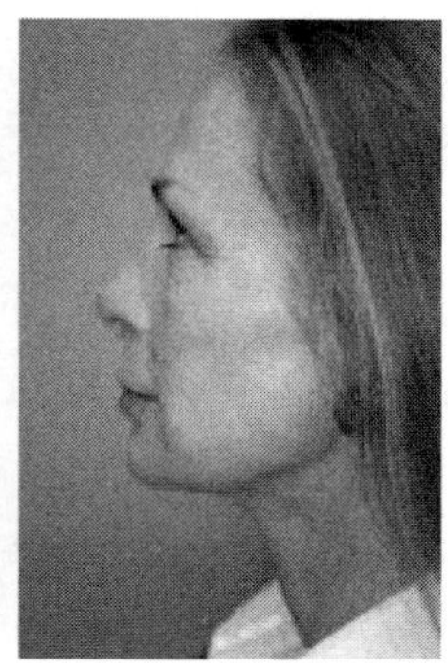

BEFORE   FIGURE 10-1A   AFTER
ENRICHED CELL ASSISTED LIPOTRANSFER (ECAL)
ACTUAL PATIENT

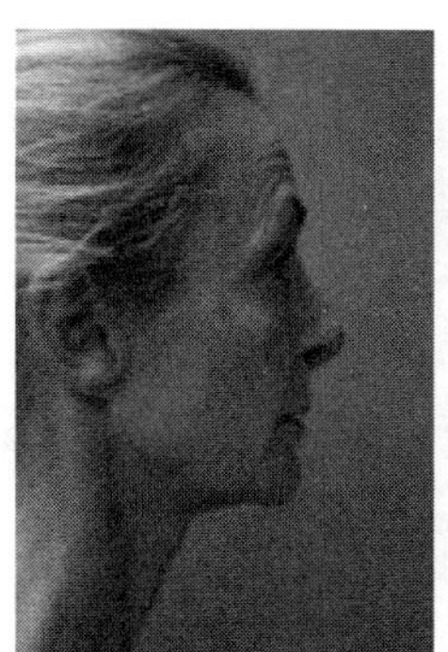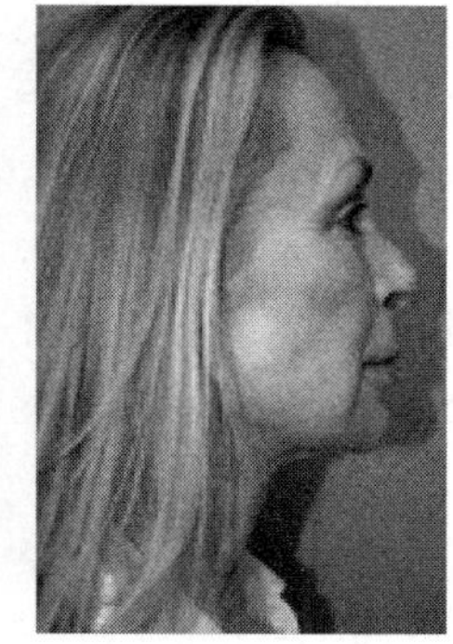

BEFORE   FIGURE 10-1B   AFTER

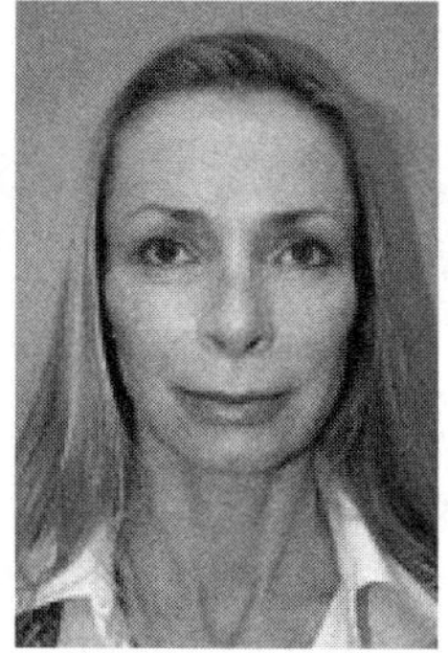

FIGURE 10-1C   AFTER

Rejuva-Lift® ECAL Breast Augmentation

Rejuva-Lift ECAL Breast Augmentation is a unique combination of liposuction and natural breast augmentation. Many candidates fear a reaction to the foreign implants used in breast augmentation. Breast enlargement through fat transfer is an excellent alternative to traditional breast implants.

This fat-transfer procedure involves extracting fat cells containing growth factors and transferring them after the fat has been removed.

Patients desiring a modest increase of one or two cup sizes are ideal candidates for ECAL Breast Augmentation.

Previously, grafting fat for breast augmentation caused calcification and scarring, visible on mammograms, and often misdiagnosed as malignancy. The Rejuva-Lift technique results in minimal calcification and scarring. Additionally, advances in mammography screening technology now help radiologists differentiate between fat-grafting changes and malignancy, with a high degree of accuracy.

ECAL can also be used to repair breast abnormalities, including deformities or implant complications, capsular contracture, rippling, or inadequate soft tissue coverage.

The 23-year-old woman in Figure 10-2 wanted to increase her breasts by one cup size. Her breasts are fuller now, and more symmetrical.

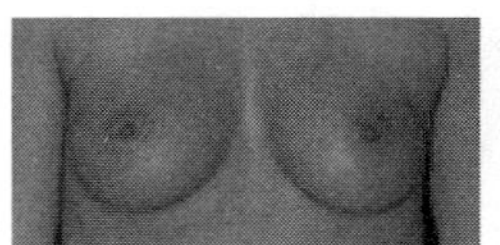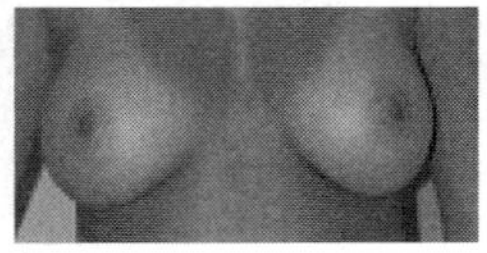

BEFORE   FIGURE 10-2   AFTER
ACTUAL PATIENT

Plasma Lipo

Plasma Lipo® is an exciting new generation of liposuction. It's a plasma ray-based procedure, developed in Japan, and involves the injection of Platelet Rich Plasma (PRP*). Figure 10-3 shows a typical Plasma Lipo unit. I was instrumental in the development of this procedure, and the first physician in the US to use it. *TO BE CONSIDERED PRP, THE PLATELET COUNT MUST BE AT LEAST 4X THE BASELINE COUNT.

What is Platelet Rich Plasma?

Platelet Rich Plasma, commonly called PRP, is processed blood plasma composed of highly concentrated platelets (shown in Figure 10-3). These platelets have been found to specialize in healing injuries to the body. Platelets also contain natural growth factors.

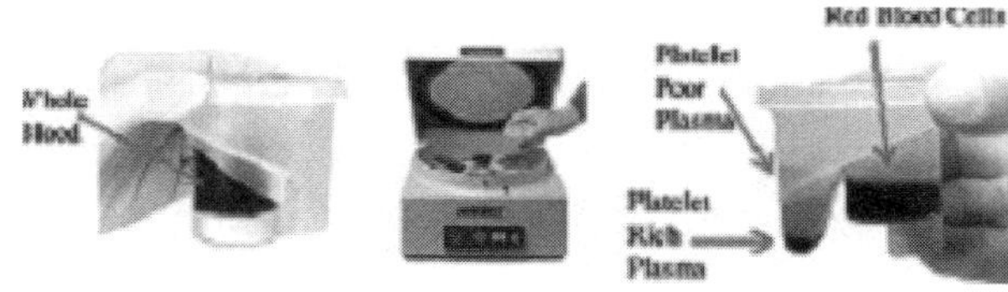

FIGURE 10-3
PLASMA LIPO PROCESS

Plasma Lipo's energy is concentrated on the end of the fiber wand (for a 360-degree attack on fat cells). A traditional lipo wand is shown in Figure 10-4 on the left, with the Plasma Lipo broadband light shown in the photo next to it.

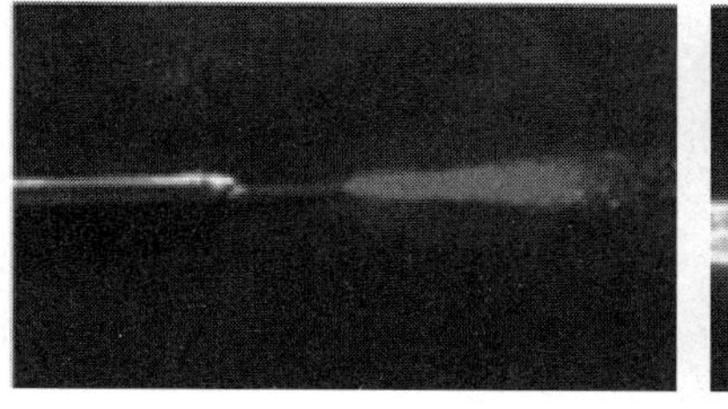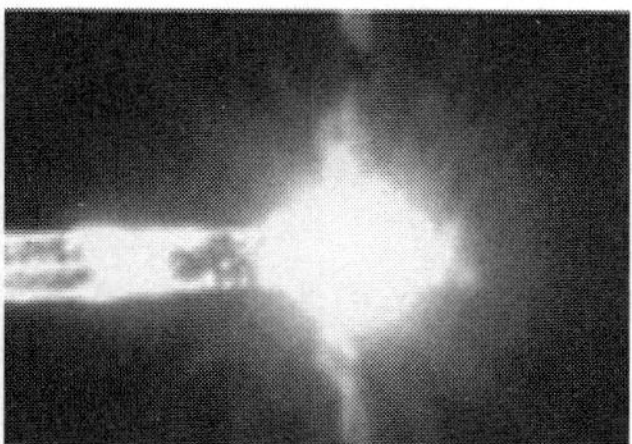

FIGURE 10-4
LASER LIPO WAND COMPARED TO PLASMA LIPO WAND

Plasma Lipo technology makes it possible to pinpoint target areas more accurately than with other laser liposuction techniques. In fact, it's been shown to be as effective in liquefying and removing fat as other lipo procedures, but requires a much lower temperature to melt fat. Consequently, there have been no reports of tissue burns.

The broadband light source also encompasses the entire spectrum of light — from 550nm to 1100nm.

Plasma Lipo has been especially effective when used to improve gynecomastia in men, and in female breast reduction, where the tissue is more fibrous and difficult to treat.

The procedure involves drawing blood (like for a blood test) then centrifuging it for about 8 minutes to separate the red blood cells from the plasma parts. See Figure 10-5. The rich platelets are then extracted and injected into the skin under a topical local anesthesia. The entire process and injection takes approximately 45 minutes to 1 hour.

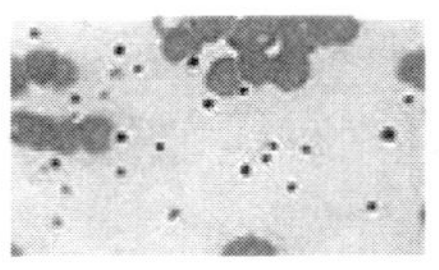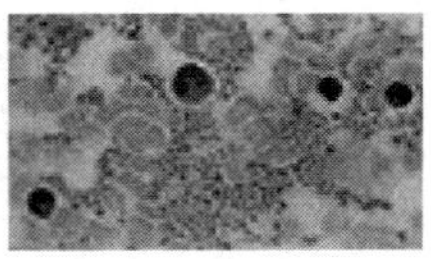

FIGURE 10-5

NORMAL PLATELET COUNT   CONCENTRATED PLATELET COUNT

Plasma Lipo is safe for areas of the body not previously treatable by traditional liposuction: face, around the eyes, chin, neck, the backs of the hands and arms, ankles, and even the calves.

Finally, Plasma Lipo can increase skin elasticity by boosting the production of collagen through the thermal action of its plasma ray.

In Conclusion

LIPOSUCTION TECHNOLOGY HAS advanced at a dizzying rate since the first crude cannulas were used to extract fat. The procedure left unsightly scars, was extremely painful, and required extensive recovery.

But the exciting possibilities of liposuction made it impossible to ignore, and once the procedure became affordable for more than just the "rich and famous", it took off like wild fire, and in every country in the world.

On the cutting edge of research into better, quicker, safer, less-invasive instruments and procedures, the United States offers a proving ground for both domestic and foreign companies hoping to build a "better mousetrap".

I have participated in researching liposuction procedures since I was first introduced to it. I'm intrigued by the latest in technology; my chosen field of liposculpture has offered me a front-row seat to watch improvements unfold. My participation in testing products and then instructing others in their use has been extremely gratifying.

I hope that this book has had a two-fold impression on you. First, that liposuction and its procedures have become clear in case you're considering liposculpture. You've been given the tools to choose a practitioner as well as the appropriate surgery.

Secondly, I hope you've gained respect for the research and technology that have resulted in what we enjoy today as the best medical care in the world.

We truly are experiencing the most profound acceleration in medical discoveries, improvements, and a coming together world-wide to tackle the questions to which, until now, there have been no answers.

Let's hope that, as one people living on this planet, we continue a respectful and productive dialog that results in even more medical miracles in the future.

Dr. Schafer's Bio

Jeffry B. Schafer, MD, FRSM, is a fully-trained Cosmetic & Reconstructive Surgeon, in practice since 1973. Along with his many years of experience in cosmetic surgery, he has 25 years of liposculpture experience.

Dr. Schafer was a former staff physician with Scripps Clinic and Research Institute in La Jolla. He was a clinical instructor at the University of Alabama's School of Medicine. Dr. Schafer also taught at the University of California at San Diego.

He is an integral part of the San Diego community. Dr. Schafer has been a board member of *Mainly Mozart,* the *San Diego Opera*, and *Partners against Crime.*

Dr. Schafer feels strongly about giving back to the community and is a supporter of the Salvation Army, numerous children's charities, and has been involved in the *Spirit of Caring Mobile Healthcare Clinic* in Chula Vista, California.

He has volunteered his plastic and reconstructive skills for the Rotary Foundation's *Thousand Smiles* in Mexico.

Dr. Schafer was awarded fellowships at King's College of the University of London, England, and the Armed Forces Institute of Pathology at Walter Reed Hospital, Washington, D.C.

Dr. Jeffry B. Schafer has been called the *"Father of Modern Laser Liposuction."* As a Cynosure Center of Excellence, his office has mentored over 120 physicians and nurse trainers in the field of laser lypolysis.

He developed the method of *Superficial Skin Tightening* and the concept of measuring skin temperature to ensure safe and accurate results during liposculpture procedures.

Dr. Schafer was instrumental in developing a protocol in the use of *SlimLipo,* introduced by Palomar Technologies. Due in part to his extensive contribution of teaching guidelines and evaluations, his practice received a *Center of Excellence* award from Palomar Technologies.

Dr. Schafer was the first physician in the US to purchase the *body jet®* liposuction system, and was showcased on *"The Doctors"* television program, demonstrating this new technology.

He was also one of the first physicians in the United States to successfully perform *Cell-Assisted Lipotransfer* of fat cells containing Stem Cells.